PARTNERSHIP WORKING IN PUBLIC HEALTH

David J. Hunter and Neil Perkins

First published in Great Britain in 2014 by

Policy Press
University of Bristol
Sixth Floor, Howard House
Queen's Avenue
Clifton
Bristol BS8 1SD
UK
Tel +44 (0)117 331 4054
Fax +44 (0)117 331 4093
e-mail pp-info@bristol.ac.uk
www.policypress.co.uk

North American office:
Policy Press
c/o The University of Chicago Press
1427 East 60th Street
Chicago, IL 60637, USA
t: +1 773 702 7700
f: +1 773-702-9756
e:sales@press.uchicago.edu
www.press.uchicago.edu

British Library Cataloguing in Publication Data
A catalogue record for this book is available from the British Library.

Library of Congress Cataloging-in-Publication Data
A catalog record for this book has been requested.

ISBN 978 1 44730 131 8 paperback
ISBN 978 1 44730 132 5 hardcover

Cover design by Qube Design Associates, Bristol
Printed and bound in Great Britain by CPI Group
(UK) Ltd,
Croydon, CR0 4YY The Policy Press uses environmentally
responsible print partners

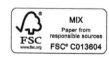

Contents

List of tables and boxes

Tables

Boxes

List of abbreviations

CCG   Clinical Commissioning Group
CMO   Chief Medical Officer
DCLG   Department for Communities and Local Government
DPH   Director of Public Health
HAZ   Health Action Zone
HImP   Health Improvement Programme
HLC   Healthy Living Centre
HWB   Health and Wellbeing Board
IDeA   Improvement and Development Agency
IOM   Institute of Medicine
JHWS   Joint Health and Wellbeing Strategy
JSNA   Joint Strategic Needs Assessment
LA   Local Authority
LAA   Local Area Agreement
LGA   Local Government Association
LGID   Local Government Improvement and Development
LSP   Local Strategic Partnership
NDC   New Deal for Communities
NHS   National Health Service
NHSCB   National Health Service Commissioning Board
NHSS   National Healthy School Standard
NICE   National Institute for Health and Care Excellence
NIHR   National Institute for Health Research
ODPM   Office of the Deputy Prime Minister
OECD   Organisation of Economic Co-operation and
         Development
PCG   Primary Care Group
PCT   Primary Care Trust
PHE   Public Health England
RCN   Royal College of Nursing
RTPI   Royal Town Planning Institute
TPP   Total Place Pilot
WHO   World Health Organization

Acknowledgements

This book has been some years in the making. Its origins go back to 2007 and the completion of a scoping study of the public health system in England commissioned by the National Institute for Health Research Service Delivery and Organisation (NIHR SDO) programme – renamed and relaunched as the Health Services & Delivery Research programme in 2012. This resulted in a successful bid to undertake a study of public health partnerships to complement the work on health and social care partnerships. While the structures associated with partnerships continue to change and evolve, there remain enduring aspects about the way in which they operate, which we have sought to draw out and emphasise in this book. In this way, we intend that the book should enjoy a longer shelf life than is usual for an account of contemporary developments in public health policy.

Various people have been associated in one way or another with this project at particular stages in its journey to publication. We are grateful to the NIHR SDO programme and, in particular, to Stephen Peckham, who was academic adviser to the SDO at the time of the research on which much of the book is based, for their support and encouragement throughout.

Others who were directly engaged with the research conducted at Durham University at various stages were, in order of involvement, Katherine Smith, Clare Bambra, Linda Marks, Kerry Joyce, Tim Blackman and Bob Hudson. They assisted with either the gathering of data, the undertaking of the systematic literature review or the offering of advice and comments on working papers and draft reports. We also received invaluable support and encouragement from Liam Hughes and Trevor Hopkins, who were both at the time based at the Healthy Communities programme run by the Improvement and Development Agency (IDeA) based at the Local Government Association. The programme and IDeA were disbanded some years ago but both did much to illuminate partnership working and the challenges and paved the way for the Health and Wellbeing Boards introduced in England in April 2013, which were intended to be a different kind of partnership drawing on the insights provided by our and other research.

Christine Jawad and Gill McGowan provided administrative support at various stages of the project for which we are most grateful.

In producing this book, we are also indebted to many others with whom we have had contact over the years and who have directly or indirectly contributed to the ideas and proposals expressed here. But we are especially indebted to those in our research study sites who gave so freely of their time and helped us understand the nature of partnership working. We hope at least some of them will find time in their busy lives to dip into the book and that it might help them in their future partnership work, as well as repay our debt to them.

Finally, all the views expressed in what follows remain entirely our own and are not necessarily shared by the NIHR, Department of Health or anyone else.

David J. Hunter and Neil Perkins
September 2013

About the authors

David J. Hunter is Professor of Health Policy and Management and Director of the Centre for Public Policy and Health, School of Medicine, Pharmacy and Health at Durham University, and a Wolfson Fellow in the Wolfson Research Institute for Health and Wellbeing. He is also Deputy Director of Fuse, the Centre for Translational Research in Public Health. He is a non-executive director of the National Institute for Health and Care Excellence (NICE). His research interests include public health policy and its implementation, prioritisation of investment and disinvestment decisions in public health commissioning in the new public health system in England, health system reform and getting knowledge into practice. He has published widely in books and journals. He is a special advisor to WHO Europe on its new health strategy, Health 2020, and accompanying European Action Plan for Strengthening Public Health Capacities and Services.

Neil Perkins is currently a Research Associate at the University of Manchester engaged in a study focusing upon the ongoing development and impact of Clinical Commissioning Groups and what value clinicians bring to commissioning. Prior to this he worked at the Centre for Public Policy and Health, Durham University, where he was engaged in a research study with Professor Hunter exploring the impact of public health partnerships in affecting public health outcomes and health inequalities, upon which this book is based. Previously, he worked on a three-year study commissioned by the Department of Health on the impact of partnership working in safeguarding vulnerable adults from abuse. Neil's research interests include partnership working in health and social care, poverty, social exclusion, 'race' and community development. Recent publications have focused on partnership working in public health and the role of partnerships in safeguarding vulnerable adults from abuse.

Series editors' foreword

Health systems are changing rapidly in response to new threats to population health from lifestyle diseases, long-term conditions and the global effects of climate change and sustainable development. Public health as a set of skills to improve health and with its focus on the health of communities rather than individuals is at the forefront of current health and health care policy and practice. In England, public health is going through a major reorganisation with local public health functions now returned to local authorities after nearly 40 years of being part of the National Health Service (NHS) and a new national public health service – Public Health England. The new organisational architecture introduced by the Health and Social Care Act 2012 has given rise to substantial uncertainty about roles and responsibilities in the new system and created a new context for developing working relationships and partnerships. While the changes have been broadly welcomed, developing the new public health system places enormous challenges on those who will lead it and also those people working within it.

This series of books on public health policy and practice aims to strengthen and add to the knowledge base for UK public health and address gaps in evidence and existing practice skills. The series has its roots in the publication of the Wanless Report (Wanless, 2004), the Cooksey Report (Cooksey, 2006) and a programme of research funded through the National Institute of Health Research (NIHR) Service Delivery and Organisation (SDO) Programme – now called the Health Services and Delivery Research programme. Cooksey identified the SDO Programme as filling an 'R&D market gap' and, therefore, of fundamental importance to the NHS (Cooksey, 2006). Following publication of the Cooksey Report, the Department of Health published *Best Research for Best Health* (DH, 2006) and the government specifically highlighted the need for the SDO Programme to commission research on public health service delivery and organisation. The SDO Programme initially commissioned Professor David Hunter to undertake a review of the state of the public health system in England in terms of its structure, capacity and skills, and the likely impact of the current changes in policy in health and local government on the public health system and their implications for its future design and effectiveness (Hunter et al, 2010). The results of this review formed the background to the commissioning of further research that addressed four key areas: governance and incentives for public health at a local level; workforce; evaluating models of public health delivery; and approaches to public and community involvement in public health – reflecting concerns raised in the Wanless Report. While commissioned in 2008 the results of this programme of research have clear implications for the development of public health services in the future. The subject of this book – public health partnerships – is perhaps of particular relevance given the developing public health system in England with its emphasis on new forms and approaches to partnership working.

This book is the third in a series that explores issues relevant to the delivery and organisation of public health. Further books are planned to examine commissioning public health, and public health in general practice. Each text presents the findings of projects commissioned by SDO (now NIHR HS&DR programme). However, it is hoped that further books will be published drawing on the work of the five UKRC Public Health Research Centres of Excellence and also the NIHR School for Public Health Research established in 2012.

The need for good-quality evidence on how to organise and deliver effective public health interventions and programmes remains a high priority. For national and local policy makers addressing new public health problems and developing effective measures for current problems raises key questions about funding, governance, the workforce, evidence of effectiveness and, increasingly, ethics.

An overarching theme in contemporary public health is the need for people to work together. The notion of collaboration and partnerships between agencies, professionals, communities and individuals is fundamental to policy for multidisciplinary public health. This book is a timely examination of this increasingly important and complex area. Who needs to work together and how can they do it most effectively? This book examines the way that concepts of collaboration and partnership are embedded within public health policy and practice. It looks at the nature of these partnerships and considers their development in the UK context and the different forms they take. The need for partnership can be seen to arise from the recognition that there are many factors which contribute to public health. In fact, this was an explicit element of the Alma Ata Declaration, where collaboration is one of the key pillars of primary health care. Collaboration was also a key element of the Health for All approach promoted by the World Health Organisation during the 1980s and subsequently reaffirmed in its current European health strategy and policy framework, *Health 2020* (WHO, 2012). Public health encompasses a diverse range of activities undertaken by a variety of actors (different government departments and agencies, professionals, private organisations, community groups, families and so on), and hence gives rise to the notion that public health is everyone's business. While the need for involving a range of agencies, and individuals, in public health has long been acknowledged (in both policy and practice) the current government has made significant shifts towards trying to co-ordinate local public health action by embedding formal public health responsibilities within local authorities. The government has also continued the emphasis on multidisciplinary and multi-organisational approaches to public health, and in England has supported new approaches to tackling public health issues, such as Whole Place Community Budgets (HM Government/LGA, 2013).

As Hunter and Perkins argue, the range of public health problems is vast and spans activities that address individual lifestyles to global health issues such as pandemics and food security. They argue that this presents particular challenges for defining public health and public health systems and represents the contested space of public health. This is the context for public health partnerships addressed in this book. Following a discussion of the scope of public health, the book explores theories of partnership and examines the literature on what makes for a successful partnership. This is an important contribution to our understanding, since most discussions of partnership in public health do not fully address key concepts and theories but rather take partnership as a necessary approach for successful public health. This book provides the foundations for such a view but one that is firmly and thoroughly underpinned by analysing the literature on the role and impacts of partnership. However, the key strength of this book is the reporting of recent research on partnerships in England. Two chapters provide an analysis of the practice of partnerships from the perspective of those managing the public health system and then from a front-line practitioner perspective. The research reported here contributes to a new emphasis in public health research, and in particular, discussions about how public health is organised. The final chapter draws together the key research findings and sets these in the context of the new English arrangements for public health. The development of new structures and roles, such as the key role of Health and Wellbeing Boards, is discussed, drawing on evidence from the research and from that provided to the House of Commons Communities and Local Government Committee's inquiry on public health (House of Commons Communities and Local Government Committee, 2013).

The authors explore issues relating to policy and practice including commissioning, new public health structures and roles – nationally and locally – and how local politics contribute to the balancing of local and national priorities. In this sense the book sets the parameters for ongoing debates about the role and nature of public health partnerships and provides a new research agenda for examining the English public health system and newly developing partnerships. Ultimately the strength of the book lies in the combination of evidence drawn from the international literature and the detailed case study research undertaken within the SDO-funded research project. There are clear lessons for practice and for those charged with developing, supporting and leading public health in the UK.

Professor Stephen Peckham
Centre for Health Services Studies, University of Kent

Professor David J. Hunter
Centre for Public Policy and Health, Durham University
August 2013

References

Cooksey, D. (2006) *A review of UK health research funding*, London: HM Treasury.

Department of Health (2006) *Best research for best health: a new national health research strategy*, London: Department of Health.

HM Government/LGA (Local Government Association) (2013) *Local public service transformation: a guide to Whole Place Community Budgets*, London: LGA.

House of Commons Communities and Local Government Committee. (2013) *The role of local authorities in health issues*, Eighth report of session 2012–13, HC 694, London: The Stationery Office.

Hunter, D.J., Marks, L. and Smith, K.E. (2010) *The public health system in England*. Bristol: Policy Press.

Wanless, D. (2004) *Securing good health for the whole population, final report*, London: Department of Health.

WHO (World Health Organization) (2013) *Health 2020*, Copenhagen: WHO.

ONE

Introduction

Little is currently known about public health partnerships, despite the fact that collaborative working is a key competency of public health practice and partnerships are still high on the policy agenda. This book draws on primary research reviewing public health partnerships, as well as on other research on partnership working more broadly. Our purpose is to establish how successful partnerships are in contributing to improved health and well-being outcomes. It is an under-explored topic in the academic literature and our intention in writing this book is to add to the evidence base while also explaining why it is difficult in practice to estalish with much certainty the impact of partnerships on outcomes.

As Dickinson and Glasby (2010, pp 813–14) note in regard to health and social care partnerships: 'over time, a series of reviews of the partnership literature all conclude that the vast majority of research to date has focused on issues of process, not on outcomes'. It is a conclusion previously reached some years earlier by Dowling et al (2004) in their literature review of partnerships. In addition to the focus on public health partnerships and their impact on health outcomes, the book also focuses on the significance of partnerships in a policy and practice context and how partnerships have evolved to tackle key public health issues. It includes commentary and analysis on the Coalition government's extensive changes in public health introduced in April 2013, which form part of a wider programme of change affecting the National Health Service (NHS) and other public services.

Partnership working has become central to British public policy, notably since the late 1990s. Its appeal lies in the fact that few challenges facing government at both national and local levels fall neatly within the confines of a single department or organisation. This is especially true of the majority of challenges facing public health, which are cross-cutting in nature and involve several policy arenas, organisations and professional groups (Hunter et al, 2010). Partnership working is neither a new nor a recent phenomenon, but it has become more pervasive in recent years. At the same time, failures in public policy are invariably laid at the door of ineffective or malfunctioning partnerships. Paradoxically, the more important partnership working has become as a mechanism for ameliorating or solving complex problems, the less effective it appears to be. The difficulties that persist have been evident for many years but have not dampened successive governments' enthusiasm for partnerships and for regarding them as essential to the successful prosecution of a raft of policies. Indeed, partnership working is generally seen as a 'good thing' (Glasby and Dickinson, 2008). As Clarke and Glendinning (2002, p 33) observe: 'Like "community", partnership is a word of obvious virtue (what sensible person would choose conflict over collaboration?)'. Dickinson and Glasby (2010, p 820) assert that it had become almost 'heretical' to argue against the integrity of partnership working. It is only in recent years that the utility of partnerships has been questioned, especially over whether they deliver 'value for money' (Audit Commission, 2005).

Therefore, the timely focus of the research study presented in this book is on outcomes and the extent to which it is possible to ascribe any progress with improvements in health and well-being to partnership working. Establishing a causal link between partnerships and outcomes is by no means a straightforward question and we make no claims to have resolved that conundrum facing researchers.

The challenge facing research in this area is in part a consequence of the very complexity of both the problems being addressed and the nature of the partnerships themselves, which have the potential to become 'the indefinable in pursuit of the unachievable' (Powell and Dowling, 2006, p 305). Moreover, for some commentators, achieving better health outcomes may not be the sole or even primary purpose of partnerships. Douglas (2009, p 2, emphasis added), for instance, suggests that while partnership working is not an end in itself, 'it is a process and a mindset, *one outcome of which may be a better service*'.

Despite there being a sizeable literature on partnerships, their typologies and how to make them work better, there are a number of important deficits that inspired the research reported here. First, most of the research on partnerships has focused on the links between health and social care (see, among others, the published work of Hudson, Glendinning, Glasby, Dickinson). With a few notable exceptions (eg the evaluation of major initiatives such as New Deal for Communities, Health Action Zones and Healthy Living Centres), there has been little research examining those partnerships concerned with public health. This may seem surprising given that public health problems often involve precisely the kind of complex interplay of factors that single organisations may find difficult to tackle in isolation. For example, the UK Government Office for Science Foresight report (Butland et al, 2007) on the complex policy challenges posed by obesity is a good example of the rationale underpinning the presumed need to work in partnership to tackle public health concerns. Such complex policy problems are commonly known as 'wicked issues' (Rittel and Webber, 1973).

From whatever angle they are viewed, public health partnerships embrace an extensive range of diverse agencies, departments, professional groups and end users and are invariably tasked with complex, multi-level and inter-sectoral interventions for which the evidence may be partial and/or contested, or even absent altogether. In addition, the very causes of the problem are likely to be multiple and subject to differing interpretations.

A second deficit, alluded to earlier, arises in regard to the available literature on partnerships demonstrating a significant, and almost exclusive, focus on process issues rather than on outcomes. This is not to denigrate the importance of process in understanding both how partnerships work and can succeed, and in identifying those components of a successful partnership that might usefully inform other partnerships being established. But the danger in focusing only, or largely, on process lies in an implicit assumption that it is a given that partnerships are desirable and will result in better outcomes just by being. Conversely, rather less attention has been given to the significant transaction costs that partnerships incur – many are 'high maintenance' (Douglas, 2009) – and to the possibility that they may contribute less to better outcomes than is assumed, or claimed, or that there might be alternative and less costly means of achieving the same, or better, results. Echoing Dowling et al's (2004) call, the need is for research that seeks to explore the success of partnerships in effecting changes in service delivery and, if possible, to establish the subsequent effects on the health and well-being of a population. Notwithstanding the difficulties besetting such a project, the research reported here is, in part, a response to that call while making no claims to be the last word on the subject.

The public health system in England

Before we proceed to focus on public health partnerships, we need to set the scene by describing briefly the public health system in England and how this has evolved and is likely to evolve in future (for a more detailed discussion of the system and its history the reader is referred to the background text for this series by Hunter, Marks and Smith [2010]).

What is a public health system?

There is, first, a need to clarify terms and state what we mean by the public health system. There are various definitions of health systems and public health systems but we have adopted the World Health Organization (WHO) perspective on these (Marks et al, 2011a). The notion of health systems is probably best captured in the definition to be found in the Tallinn Charter (WHO, 2008, p 1, para 2):

> Within the political and institutional framework of each country, a health system is the ensemble of all public and private organisations, institutions and resources mandated to improve, maintain or restore health. Health systems encompass both personal and population services, as well as activities to influence the policies and actions of other sectors to address the social, environmental and economic determinants of health.

This definition of health systems is both wide-ranging and aspirational. It stresses the scope of health systems beyond health care and is inclusive of 'those stewardship activities that aim to influence what other sectors do when it is relevant to health, even where the primary purpose is not health' (Figueras et al, 2008, p vii). Nevertheless, it is likely that most health systems remain largely associated with, and have their origins in, health care systems, which, unlike public health systems, have relatively *clear* and circumscribed organisational boundaries. Many organisations, notably, local authorities, would be unlikely to regard or classify themselves as belonging to a health system. Anything with 'health' in the title would be deemed a matter involving medical or clinical care. Therefore, by subsuming public health systems within health systems, the range and scope of public health activities may be unintentionally narrowed. A health care system is typically focused on 'identifying and repairing health problems arising from past exposures' and does not concern itself with the inter-sectoral focus of public health or its future challenges (Graham, 2010, p 151).

The definition of a public health system is contingent on the meaning and scope of public health. In keeping with the Acheson definition of public health,'public health is the science and art of preventing disease, prolonging life and promoting health through the organised efforts of society' (Acheson, 1998, p 1). This is a very broad definition that emphasises 'whole of government' and 'whole of society' approaches. It suggests that a public health system is considered as more inclusive than a health system. However, including all and every entity and activity that may have a bearing on health as forming part of a public health system suffers from the problem of seeking to be all-encompassing. But it is only when different organisations work interactively, possibly in partnership, towards a shared objective, working as a whole, that they can be defined as working as a system (IOM, 2003).

Operationalising activities, intelligence, systems, skills and competencies for public health is consequent upon the definition of public health and what constitutes a public health problem. The range of public health problems is vast and includes, at one level, encouraging individuals to lead healthier lifestyles while, at another, tackling global health issues involving climate change, population growth, health protection against pandemics and food security. It is the gap between the challenges and the activities of public health practice to tackle them that constitutes the arena in which many of the debates over definitions and the scope of public health activity are located and get played out. This, in turn, represents the 'contested space' of public health and the approach taken will influence a number of issues with the system, including: the breadth of a public health system and of public health partnerships within it; the integration of public health services into health care services, notably, primary care; the nature of interactions between public health systems and broader political, social, economic and cultural systems; and the future orientation of the public health workforce and public health systems (Marks et al, 2011a). Finding an optimal balance between these issues will not be resolved through technical arguments or agreements over definitions. These are unlikely to hold in any case since many of the key issues are inherently political and value-based and subject to continuous negotiation.

Therefore, rather than attempt to solve the conundrum of what is a public health system once and for all through a possibly futile search for a universal definition of such a system, Hunter, Marks and Smith (2010) argue that a networked approach is more likely to better reflect the diversity of organisations and sectors with a bearing on specific issues that pose a threat to population health, or, conversely, may serve to enhance it. The precise dimensions and boundaries of a public health system will therefore vary according to the particular health issue being addressed and the effectiveness of the system will depend on the active engagement of all relevant organisations.

In adopting such a flexible perspective on the public health system, four approaches may be considered in framing public health systems and their constituent parts (Marks et al, 2011a). These may overlap in practice. First is the public health workforce and infrastructure, which may be viewed as meeting the requirements of the three domains developed by Griffiths, Jewell and Donnelly (2005):

- *Health improvement:* promoting healthy lifestyles and healthy environments and encompassing issues of inequality and the wider social determinants of health.
- *Health protection:* protecting people from specific threats to their health, including such activities as immunisation and vaccination, screening, injury prevention, control of infectious diseases, and emergency planning.
- *Health service improvement:* bringing an evidence-based population perspective to planning, commissioning and evaluating services and interventions to ensure that they are effective, high-quality, safe and accessible, and supporting clinical governance.

These three domains are not discrete entities, but overlap and are interdependent. Nevertheless, each entails a sizeable remit and involves a varied mix of skills and expertise. For instance, health promotion demands an exceptional range of competencies, as well as cross-government policy and joined-up management at various levels, an ability to work in partnership with a diverse range of agencies and professionals (each displaying its own values, beliefs and interests), and the skills to support and strengthen community action. The other two domains are just as complex in their own ways and a great deal of coordination is required in those situations where all three domains are involved. This applies in regard to many contemporary public health issues such as teenage pregnancy or alcohol misuse, for example, where each of the three domains might have a contribution to make in framing the actions required and in identifying the stakeholders who need to be engaged in constructing and delivering them.

A second approach to framing public health systems may be described as an inclusive approach, as set out by the Institute of Medicine (IOM, 2003). It applies where a public health system is not limited to those with a formal role in improving health, but reflects those organisations and groups that have an influence on health and that may need to work in concert for health issues to be appropriately addressed. This approach includes communities, the health care delivery system, employers and business, the media, academia, and the governmental public health infrastructure. The inclusive approach subscribes to the importance of inter-sectoral approaches in the context of the influences on health. It also reflects an awareness of the impact on health of non-health sectors and the limitations of medical care in isolation in promoting population health. Such an approach is reflected in the notions of 'healthy public policy' and 'ecological public health' (Lang and Rayner, 2012). It also underpins the European Union (EU) commitment to Health in All Policies (HiAP) (Stahl et al, 2006). Lang and Rayner (2012) express the challenge as follows: '21st century ecological public health must address the inherent complexity of shaping factors across what we call the four dimensions of existence'. These are: (a) the material dimension; (b) the biological dimension; (c) the cultural dimension; and (d) the social dimension. They continue: 'public health in the 21st century requires policies and actions to engage in all four dimensions of existence to be most effective' (Lang and Rayner, 2012).

The third approach is an extension of the IOM approach but with a greater focus on identifying and clarifying in a proactive manner the roles of a wide range of organisations in addressing specific health issues and developing system-wide action to address their complex causes and consequences. An example of such an approach is the UK Government Office for Science Foresight report on obesity, which described the problem as centring on an obesogenic environment. This framed the challenge as a societal one demanding a societal response (Butland et al, 2007). The problem cannot be solved by single or simple solutions, such as modifying individual lifestyles, but demands a multifaceted and multi-levelled response that tackles the causes of the causes. While the formal public health system might initiate action, it need not do so exclusively. A range of other groups and organisations is likely to be involved, including those representing the food and drinks industries. The challenge would be to identify those groups and bodies that would need to work together at various levels in a connected way (ie as a system) to address public health concerns.

Fourth, and finally, in terms of framing a public health system is mobilising support and action across different sectors to provide a counter-response to emerging threats to population health. Here, the focus is on an advocacy approach in order to put health issues firmly on the policy agendas of governments, business and others at various levels.

Marks et al (2011b) consider that an effective public health system should incorporate all four elements, building on the core activities suggested by the first approach but drawing on the others as appropriate. A key challenge for public health practitioners and advocates for public health is to engage those organisations and groups whose principal interest may not be obviously or explicitly health-related, and who would therefore fall outside health systems as described earlier, but whose actions nonetheless have a significant impact on health in its widest sense. At the same time, it remains the case that even within traditional health care systems, there is considerable scope for encouraging and fostering more upstream interventions concerned with health promotion and disease prevention. In the UK, the 'making every contact count' initiative is designed to do precisely this, although whether it is sufficient to sustain good health remains uncertain.

Central to our discussion, though, public health work implies collective action and that invariably requires some form of partnership working. The strength of a public health system can be gauged by the extent to which relevant groups work effectively together on specific issues in a flexible, organic and customised manner, rather than in a mechanistic or rigid way, whereby all those organisations with an impact on health are brought together to act in ways that are not always clear or achievable given their competing interests, values or resource differentials. This issue goes to the heart of what makes for effective public health partnerships, which is, of course, the subject of this book. Before we turn to such matters, however, we need first to describe briefly the nature of the public health system in England and how it has evolved in recent decades in order to set the scene for what follows in the remainder of the book.

The evolving public health system in England

Until 1974, responsibility for the public health function in England lay with local government. However, during the upheaval in the NHS in 1974, when it underwent its first major reorganisation, the lead responsibility for public health moved to the NHS, with public health doctors attached to the new health authorities. This situation maintained until April 2013, when the Coalition government announced in 2010 that public health should return to local government, where, it claimed, it more naturally belonged. Local government did not lose all its public health functions, however, since environmental health remained under its control.

Despite the NHS having the lead role for public health for over almost 40 years, the position was never regarded by many in local government or elsewhere as a settled one. Various recurring themes, tensions and schisms marked the history of the public health function during this period. Among these has been continuing debate over the optimal location of the public health function and whether it has been well-served by being located in the NHS since 1974. Many believe that it has not, especially since the emergence of the movement known as 'the new public health' in the late 1970s, which sought to broaden the discourse around health and the factors contributing to it, as well as tackle the complex challenges it posed. Other recurring tensions included: the focus on the social determinants of health versus attempts to influence individual lifestyles; the nature and conceptualisation of the public health workforce in terms of both capacity and capability and the skills required for the varied and complex responsibilities it had acquired; the balance between 'upstream' public health interventions on the one hand and 'downstream' health care services on the other, which for the most part were deemed to have a limited role in improving health; and the nature and scope of the public health system, which we have discussed already but which remained an issue in the light of the other tensions identified.

Perhaps somewhat paradoxically, having moved most major public health responsibilities from local government to the NHS in 1974, the period since then has been marked by various attempts to ensure that responsibility for public health was shared between agencies and across jurisdictions, with a truly multidisciplinary workforce being the goal. Most of these attempts, including the introduction in 2007 of joint Director of Public Health (DPH) posts operating between the NHS and local government, have been patchy, uneven and generally found wanting (Hunter, 2008a). It is in this context that the rise of public health partnerships occurred and has become something of an industry in itself.

The chief criticism of the move of public health to the NHS under the label 'community medicine' was that before long, most community physicians became victims of the managerialist revolution, which, starting with the 1974 reorganisation, gripped the NHS and has been much in evidence ever since. Community physicians were unclear as to where their primary responsibility lay – was it to the management of health services, or to the analysis of health problems and health needs and how these might best be met (Lewis, 1986). Though many working in public health were concerned about the downstream focus of much of their work within the NHS, others accepted it as the price to be paid for securing a seat at the top table when it came to deciding priorities and making resource allocation decisions. However, for all that, community medicine failed to achieve the status desired by its architects – it never achieved parity with other clinical specialties, especially hospital-based ones – and recruitment declined.

Concerns about the loss of public health from local government should not be mistaken for the loss of a 'golden age' in public health. No one, it seems, considered the Medical Officer of Health (MOH) model in local government to be above criticism. The best MOHs were key figures in their communities and used their position to advance a community health agenda (Gorsky, 2007). However, to suggest that 'an enormously vigorous public health system' was in some way neutered by the move of the function to the NHS is not a sustainable position to adopt (Lewis, 1986, p 163); other systemic forces were also at work, which undermined and marginalised public health and contributed to low morale and under-resourcing. Chief among these forces were: first, the increasing bias towards hospitals in the NHS despite the NHS having been established to promote health and not merely tend to the sick once ill; and, second, the attenuation of local authority powers, which made it difficult to develop and progress its public health role. Albeit in different contexts, both these systemic forces remain evident and merely relocating public health back to local government, as the Coalition government has sought to do, is unlikely in itself to redress the power imbalance between health and health care. As we caution later in the book in Chapter Six, it would be a cruel paradox indeed if just when public health returns to local government, the new structures being established to advance the cause get hijacked or derailed by issues within the NHS that largely affect health care services. It would not be the first time that this has happened, and local authorities are likely to be especially sensitive to such issues affecting as they do the range and type of health services available and the intense local politics accompanying them should they be up for reconfiguration, merger or, worse, closure. With public finances being severely squeezed, the pressures on hospital services in particular and the need for changes in their configuration have never been greater.

As noted, the specialty of community medicine underwent something of an identity crisis when it was established given the lack of status accorded it and the absence of any clarity as to its proper role. This gave rise to an inquiry led by the then Chief Medical Officer (CMO) for England, Donald Acheson. Completed in 1988, its upshot was the need for a multidisciplinary approach to public health, although the specialty would continue to be led by medically qualified professionals with others from other backgrounds performing supportive roles. The specialty was also renamed 'public health medicine'.

Although in some ways an improvement on what had existed previously, it was not long before significant tensions surfaced over inequalities of opportunities for non-medical staff working within the new system. This resulted in some of those working in public health establishing their own ad hoc networks (Evans and Knight, 2006). But none of these enjoyed professional recognition and there were no proper agreed career structures for non-medical public health staff. The focus of training and development was firmly on those who were medically qualified. Frustrations mounted and the Faculty of Public Health Medicine became the crucible in which they were played out.

The early 1990s witnessed a growing acceptance, at least in policy terms, that the public health function should not be defined by, or restricted to, a medical specialty (Jacobson et al, 1991). It was probably the result of an inevitable and pragmatic realisation that the status quo was no longer sustainable, and a response to increasingly vociferous calls to develop a multidisciplinary workforce (Evans and Knight, 2006). It was some years hence, however, before real progress occurred and it took a change of government, a new CMO and a critical House of Commons Health Select Committee report to get action. The new CMO had inherited from his predecessor a review of the public health workforce with a view to strengthening public health (Department of Health, 2001). This report had quite a lot to say about the wider public health workforce and the need to move away from an almost exclusive focus on public health as a clinical specialty. It identified three broad categories of people comprising the public health workforce:

- *Specialists:* consultants in public health medicine and specialists in public health who work at a strategic or senior management level or at a senior level of scientific expertise to influence the health of the population or of a selected community.
- *Public health practitioners:* those who spend a major part, or all, of their time in public health practice – for example, health visitors and school nurses.
- *Wider public health:* most people, including managers, who have a role in health improvement and reducing health inequalities although they may not recognise this themselves, including teachers, social workers, local business leaders, transport engineers, town planners, housing officers, regeneration managers and so on.

There were other developments around this time. One of them took its cue from the government's public health White Paper, *Saving lives: our healthier nation* (Secretary of State for Health, 1999), which announced a number of initiatives intended to help develop a genuinely multidisciplinary public health function, including the establishment of the post of specialist in public health, which was to be of equivalent status in independent practice to medically qualified consultants in public health medicine and allow non-clinical public health specialists to become directors of public health (Secretary of State for Health, 1999). The following year, in 2000, the Secretary of State for Health at the time, Alan Milburn, gave the London School of Economics and Political Science annual health lecture in which he called on those involved in public health to end 'lazy thinking and occupational protectionism' and 'take public health out of the ghetto' (Milburn, 2000). As if in response to these rather searing criticisms, in the same year, the Faculty of Public Health Medicine agreed that membership of the Faculty should be opened to candidates from disciplines other than medicine and, in 2003, finally dropped 'Medicine' from its title.

Further pressure on the public health community came with the Wanless review of public health (Wanless, 2004). Commissioned by the government of the day in 2003, specifically, the Prime Minister, Secretary of State for Health and Chancellor, the review was a follow-up to the earlier commissioned review of health trends and the long-term financial and resource needs of the NHS to 2022 (Wanless, 2002). The focus of the 2004 review was on prevention and the wider determinants of health in England since these had been key themes in the first review and the government wanted an update of the challenges involved in turning the NHS into a truly 'health' service, especially as these affected public health. Wanless questioned the cost-effectiveness of action and called for more rigorous and long-term implementation of sustainable solutions often lacking due to poor public health information and an evidence base. To address these issues, he went on to state:

> Adequate workforce capacity will need to be created with appropriately broad skill mixes. Because more of the activity will be concerned with monitoring, interpreting data, identifying risk, educating people and motivating them to change behaviour, the required mix of skills will change. (Wanless, 2004, p 9)

All of these developments chimed with the government's drive to increase public health workforce capacity, accompanied by moves to ensure that the workforce become more multidisciplinary in nature. To assist with strengthening the wider public health workforce, the UK Voluntary Register for Public Health Specialists was established in 2003 to help assure the quality of the new breed of non-clinical specialists.

Despite important and impressive progress having been made to open up public health to a wider range of competencies and expertise, elements of medical hegemony remain and are never far from discussions about the quality of public health practitioners and whether this has been impaired by the move to expand the workforce. For example, Wright (2007, p 219) claims that medical resistance, which remains alive, has focused on concerns about whether the route to such specialist posts open to non-medical specialists (achieved via a portfolio approach) constitutes a real equivalence to the route taken by medically qualified personnel, suggesting that it is perhaps 'an easy alternative to higher specialist training'. It is a charge that has festered to this day, breaking out most recently when the government carried out a review of the regulation of public health professionals in 2010 (Department of Health, 2010). In the words of its author, Gabriel Scally, then Regional Director for Public Health in NHS South West, the purpose of regulation was the avoidance of 'morbidity or mortality resulting from poor professional practice' (Department of Health, 2010, p 4), and, in his view, the current system was unsatisfactory and required improving in quality and clarifying. The issue has divided the public health community. The desire for statutory, in place of voluntary, regulation is suspected by supporters of the voluntary register as a move by clinicians to wrest back control of the specialty amid fears that the preponderance of non-medically qualified practitioners now entering the specialty is giving cause for concern over the maintenance of standards. Having initially deferred making a decision pending further views on the matter, in its response to the Health Committee's report, the government announced its decision to bring in statutory regulation of non-medical public health consultants to help ensure more consistent standards across the profession (Secretary of State for Health, 2012). The plan is to legislate to give the Health Professions Council responsibility for regulating this group of practitioners.

It may be no coincidence that the issue has also arisen at the very time that the lead role for public health in England is moving back to local government, with fears that this may also serve to lower standards and further reduce the number of medically qualified public health specialists. It is certainly an issue that the Health Committee took seriously in its inquiry into the public health changes (House of Commons Health Committee, 2011).

We have described the evolution of the public health system and its workforce because it provides essential background to our exploration of public health partnerships and the move of public health back to local government in England. Given the changes that have occurred, and others still to come, these cannot but be influenced by the past, and by recent history in particular. Much of the opposition to the current changes, and in particular the return of public health to local government, has come directly from public health clinicians who disagree with those who consider that the NHS has not proved to be the optimal location for the public health function (McKee et al, 2011). Their concern is that public health standards will suffer in a highly politicised environment of the kind to be found in local government and that, by its very nature, local government will encourage variation and diversity, which are not in the best interests of public health nationally if inequalities are not to widen and poor health to worsen. Allied to these concerns is a fear that the cherished independence of DPHs and their annual reports will become eroded through working in an intensely political environment within local government, where the leaders are elected members and not the officers. For many DPHs, this amounts to something of a culture shock, which may well explain why many DPH posts have become vacant and why those accustomed to an NHS setting have sought to switch to employment in Public Health England rather than have to move to local government.

It is highly likely that as the new arrangements, which we describe and assess in some detail in Chapter 6, come into being and start to bed down, tensions and power struggles that have never been fully resolved will resurface once again. The fate of future partnerships will to some degree depend upon how these struggles get played out in the context of the new structures and systems being put in place. Certainly, the history of public health partnerships hitherto, as our own research reported later shows, has not been unaffected by such tensions and disputes, which is a major, though by no means the only, reason for such constructs having for the most part failed to make the impact they could, and possibly ought to, have had.

However, other, wider factors cannot be ignored either. They have their origins in how we view organisational performance and effectiveness. The persistence of a rational, linear approach to conceptualising effective partnerships, where there is perfect clarity and agreement over roles and responsibilities, is at odds with an increasingly complex and unpredictable reality. What is required is to break free from these mind traps and think differently about the whole partnership enterprise. We explore some of the alternative approaches that might be adopted later in the book and conclude that if the new arrangements are going to make a difference and be different, then they must adopt a different way of approaching their work.

We do not think that we are being especially radical or counter-intuitive in offering these insights about alternatives as we think they actually reflect more accurately what makes for a successful partnership in practice. Paradoxically, we tend to make life more difficult for ourselves by over-organising and producing ever-more elaborate wiring diagrams to depict the perfect partnership, which deny a rather more messy reality, but one that can often produce results that make sense to those directly engaged. If the renewed commitment to localism is to mean anything, it surely has to allow for local experimentation and diversity. The problem is that the pull to the centre remains so powerful in the UK when compared with other European countries; local agencies have lost the ability to think for themselves or to seize the initiative. This is certainly true of the NHS over the years. It is hopefully less true of local government, although, even here, since most of its finance comes from central government grants, there remains a tendency to look upwards and not downwards and/or outwards to local communities.

Possibly, the real test of the changes is whether they are able to redress the powerful centrifugal forces evident within British society and encourage and make a reality of rather weaker centripetal ones. Public health requires a mix of both if the problems that it seeks to address are to be tackled effectively. Action locally is vital but can only go so far, and much of what happens at this level needs to take the form of advocacy and putting pressure on higher levels to act in ways that align with local efforts. If the new partnership arrangements can assist in squaring the circle – assisting with what can be done locally to improve health as well as acting as an advocate for change elsewhere in government – then the changes might be deemed to have been worth the considerable trouble and cost (human and financial) that have been incurred. But we will not know that for some time.

Plan of the book

The research presented in this book is located within a wider policy context that has been subject to considerable, and largely unexpected and unforeseen, change since the research was undertaken. This period of unprecedented change began with the election of the UK Coalition government in May 2010. While these developments in no way negate the findings and conclusions emanating from the research, the changing context offers opportunities both to reassess the way in which partnerships are designed and to take account of the lessons from research, such as the project reported here. The research is also placed within a broader context in respect of critically evaluating approaches to partnership working and the effectiveness of partnerships. Following this introductory chapter, the book is organised into six further chapters.

Chapter Two, drawing on the relevant literature, discusses the rationale for partnerships and presents a typology of partnerships, moving along a continuum from loose networks, through formal statutory partnerships, to integrated structures involving different agencies. Many of these arrangements impact on, and give rise to new forms of, governance. These, in turn, give rise to important issues of power and accountability in respect of how partnerships are managed and operate. Key issues surrounding defining partnerships, what makes a partnership a 'success' and what the major barriers are to partnership working are also explored.

Chapter Three reviews the extensive literature on partnerships in order to demonstrate how little is known about their impact on, and contribution to, outcomes. The first systematic review of public health partnerships and outcomes, conducted as part of the study reported here, is presented. It focuses on the key policy initiatives introduced by governments since the late 1990s to improve public health and reduce health inequalities. This was an especially fertile period of innovation in health policy, and central to a range of initiatives, notably, Health Action Zones, Health Improvement Programmes and the New Deal for Communities, was the notion of partnership working.

The next two chapters present the empirical findings from the research on which the book is based. Key to the study is the view that partnerships are regarded as integral to the pursuit of public health. *Chapter Four* considers the views of senior practitioners on the effectiveness and efficacy of public health partnerships. This grouping includes DPHs, Directors of Commissioning, Councillors and other senior public health practitioners. The research focuses upon a number of questions, including: 'What is understood by public health partnerships?'; 'Can policy goals and objectives be achieved without partnerships?'; 'What are the determinants of a "successful" or "effective" partnership?'; 'What barriers exist to partnership working?'; 'What is the impact of partnerships on health outcomes?'; and 'What issues do partnerships face in future?'.

More specifically, among public health professionals, these questions become more focused and concentrate on operational issues of partnership working, and further issues are addressed, such as:

- How effective are joint DPH posts?
- What is the impact of partnerships on joint commissioning?
- What is the role and scope of partnerships in Local Area Agreements?
- What is the evidence in regard to the impact of partnerships on outcomes?

Chapter Five seeks to ascertain the key differences in the styles of partnership working on the front line as distinct from a strategic level, and, in addition to the questions on the success and barriers to partnerships identified earlier, concentrates on the following questions:

- What are the benefits of partnerships for service users?
- What are the views of service users towards partnership working?
- How do networking and partnership-working arrangements differ from those at a strategic level?
- How 'joined up' are the partnership agendas from the strategic level to working on the front line?

Chapter Six brings the review and assessment of partnerships up-to-date by focusing on the Coalition government's changes for public health partnerships arising from the Health and Social Care Act 2012 and critically appraising these in terms of what they might mean for the future of partnership working in public health. The potential impact that the role of public health being relocated to local authorities will have on partnerships is explored, as is the impact of the establishment of Public Health England. In particular, will the reorganisation of public health and the simultaneous restructuring of the NHS, involving the abolition of Primary Care Trusts and Strategic Health Authorities, mean that partnerships are likely to become severely fractured or dismembered and will have to be reconstructed? Will the loss of 'corporate memory' – key individuals either being relocated or exiting the public health arena altogether – result in a loss of expertise in addition to the loss of 'local champions', that is, those who champion partnership working and act as a bridge between partner organisations? Will such losses actually matter if public health partnerships in the past, as our review of existing research and our own research show, were of variable quality and had patchy success at best? With the new Health and Wellbeing Boards tasked to secure partnership working between NHS services, social care and public health, what challenges and opportunities do they face? Might they succeed in breaking the mould and giving rise to new and more effective partnership forms, or will they revert to the default position of becoming crippled by a fixation on structure and governance arrangements? Or might they be captured by the priority being accorded health and social care integration at the possible expense of a focus on health prevention and well-being? Finally, with the increased emphasis on privatisation and competition with 'any qualified provider' invited to tender to provide a range of health and related services, is the cooperative and collaborative nature of partnership working at risk? Is it destined to assume a lesser role in policy and operational contexts?

Chapter Seven is the final chapter and draws the key arguments and issues together while at the same time speculating on the future of public health partnerships. Do they have one? Where might it lead?

What might public health partnerships look like in the future? What are the key priorities for such partnerships and how do they need to adapt in a much-changed policy landscape?

TWO

Theories and concepts of partnerships

Partnerships, whether of the public–public or public–private variety, have become the *sine qua non* of British public policy, especially since the late 1990s, and, as Balloch and Taylor (2001b, p 2) state of partnership working, it is 'a term that commands widespread support across the political spectrum'. However, working in partnership is not a recent phenomenon. Powell and Glendinning (2002) argue that partnerships have been a feature of public policy since the 1601 Poor Law, and Hudson et al (1999) note that in their 1909 Minority Report to the Poor Law Commission, social reformers Sidney and Beatrice Webb argued that in order to prevent poverty, different strands of policy and agencies needed to be brought together.

The journey towards partnerships becoming a common feature in public policy can be seen most clearly from the post-war period onwards. The command-and-control hierarchical approach characterised by 'Old Labour', which dominated much of the period up to the end of the 1970s as part of the post-war consensus, was seen as inadequate to tackle complex policy problems (Ling, 2002). However, the journey was not an entirely straightforward one and there were some wrong turns along the way that hindered progress. In particular, the market-driven approach of the Conservatives between 1979 and 1997 has been characterised as one that made coordination difficult due to the competitive element of policy whereby agencies were actively encouraged to compete, rather than cooperate, with one another in regard to funding and resources (Ling, 2002; Powell and Glendinning, 2002).

Although initially committed to abolishing the internal market in health, New Labour subsequently embraced, and even promoted, it under the rubric of a 'third way' (Hunter, 2008b). Of considerable appeal to its principal architect, Prime Minister Blair, the 'third way' approach was the principal driver of policy under New Labour when it formed the government in 1997 and it sought to reject both the hierarchical 'command-and-control' approach embraced by 'Old Labour' and the market-driven approach of the Conservatives, advocating instead a network or partnership approach to governance that was neither the state nor the market in their pure forms. The favoured mantra at the time was 'what works is what matters', and for New Labour, the public–private distinction was viewed as unhelpful and a brake on progress in improving the performance of public services. As Clarke and Glendinning (2002, p 33) note:

> Partnership embodies the 'betwixt and between' spirit of the Third Way, being neither a state bureaucratic system nor a market place of contending interests. As such, it expresses the non-ideological, non-dogmatic orientation of the Third Way, moving beyond the 'old' ideological commitments to the market or the state.

Partnerships were also favoured as the ideal policy mechanism to tackle those intractable policy problems that were not believed to be adequately addressed under the hierarchical or market-driven approaches. These intractable policy problems were termed 'wicked issues', which Ling (2002, p 622) describes as 'a class of problems whose causes are so complex, and whose solutions are so multi-factorial, that they require a multi-agency response'.

With the election of New Labour, a slew of policy initiatives, measures and taskforces were launched to make partnership working a reality. Prominent among them were Health Action Zones, Education Action Zones, New Deal for Communities, Sure Start and Crime and Disorder Partnerships. All these initiatives had partnership working as their central feature and also included joint strategic plans for specific clusters of services, joint funding arrangements, pooled budgets and joint service provision (Glendinning et al, 2005a). Working in partnership had also become a central requirement of funding bids, as well as consulting with communities and service users (Balloch and Taylor, 2001b). Sullivan and Skelcher estimated that there were about 5,500 individual public policy partnership bodies clustering into almost 60 types, with 75,000 board members spending some £4.3 billion in 2001/02 (cited in Powell and Dowling, 2006). Public health, with its plethora of 'wicked issues', seemed to be especially well placed when it came to demonstrating the need for partnership working.

Although they confront many of the same issues as those arising in other types of partnership, it seems a fair assumption to make that public health partnerships are more complex and long-term in their impact on health outcomes. For the most part, this is because, as already noted, they are concerned with 'wicked issues'; in the public health context, this means issues where complex interdependencies are involved, where causality is difficult to unravel or ascribe, and where outcomes are unpredictable or may have unintended consequences (Rittel and Webber, 1973; Stewart, 1998; Australian Public Service Commission, 2007). Such complex problems also go beyond the capacity of any single organisation to understand and respond to, and there is often disagreement about the causes of the problems that can make it difficult to decide whose responsibility it is. Take the example of speed humps to slow traffic and make streets in built-up areas safer. These have been popular in the UK and elsewhere but some experts argue that they are more likely to contribute to injury and death than to prevent them (Abrahamson and Freedman, 2006). The main problem is the slowing of emergency vehicles such as ambulances and fire engines. In the case of the former, speed humps have been cited as a factor in London's unusually poor survival rate for heart attack victims; in the case of fire engines, the jolt going over the humps has caused permanent spinal injury to firefighters. Also, buses with low floors to make access easier for disabled people are vulnerable to damage.

Compared with public health partnerships confronting such 'wicked issues', those partnerships operating in health and social care are comparatively straightforward. They may be complicated but not complex, with the goals they seek to achieve being reasonably clear and well-defined. It may help explain why Douglas, though under no illusions about the difficulties partnerships face, is able to view the future of partnership working in social care with some optimism. He believes that progress is evident in enough areas 'to contemplate a time when partnership working will eventually become redundant terminology because it is a way of life' (Douglas, 2009, p 227). In contrast, public health goals are invariably less clear and are often contested. For example, should the focus on tackling obesity be on children or adults or both? Should it be on tackling individual behaviour or on collective action, such as taking the food and drink industry to task for manufacturing, and/or selling cheaply, unhealthy products high in sugar, salt and fat that contribute to obesity? In addition, there is the sheer breadth of the public health function, with its focus on the so-called three domains of health promotion, health protection and health service improvement, and the multiple ways in which public health issues are conceptualised, operationalised and prioritised across various sectors (Griffiths et al, 2005; Hunter et al, 2010).

Partnership working was therefore regarded as the best, if not only, organisational mechanism fit for the task, although the reasons why it should hold such appeal remain rather obscure and may not be borne out by the available evidence. On his reading of the large and rapidly growing academic literature on partnerships of one sort or another, Pollitt draws conclusions that are less well-disposed towards them:

> The main message I draw ... [is] that 'partnership' is a very variable concept, that it is often not well-understood, and that, while it seems to work reasonably well under certain conditions, there are many situations in which it should probably not be the government's first choice of organisational form. (Pollitt, 2003, pp 57–8)

Perhaps, therefore, partnerships should not be taken at face value as axiomatically 'a good thing'.

What's in a name? Defining partnerships

On the surface, 'partnership' seems a pretty straightforward and clear-cut term, but in policy and practice, it has proven to be a somewhat elusive concept and a portmanteau term. Of course, that lack of clarity and fuzziness can sometimes suit policymakers because it lends the concept infinite flexibility and makes it more malleable in practice to suit a variety of circumstances. Certainly, in policy documents and in its usage across the policy spectrum, the term 'partnership' is diverse and diffuse, with multiple terms having been employed to describe it. 'Collaboration', 'joined-up working', 'cooperation', 'networking', 'multi-agency working', 'joint planning', 'alliance' and 'inter-organisational relations' are but just a few of the terms commonly used. Leathard argued that 'partnerships' mean all things to all people and observed that it was a 'terminological quagmire', using 52 separate terms to illustrate the point (cited in Glasby and Dickinson, 2008). Many others have also cited the imprecise definitional nature of working in partnership (see, eg, Huxham 2003; Wildridge et al, 2004; Dowling et al, 2004; Williams and Sullivan, 2009). Ling (2000, p 82) describes the partnership literature as amounting to 'methodological anarchy and definitional chaos'. This is perhaps best encapsulated by Powell and Glendinning (2002, p 2), who argue that: 'Partnership[s] risk becoming a "Humpty Dumpty" term ("When I call something a partnership, by definition it is one ...")'. Yet, as Glasby and Dickinson (2008) argue, although 'partnership' may be an imprecise term, with no agreed definition, it is the best we have.

However, a number of definitions have been constructed to capture what characterises working in partnership. The Audit Commission

(1998, p 8) used the term 'partnership' to describe a joint-working arrangement where the partners:

- are otherwise independent bodies;
- agree to cooperate to achieve a common goal;
- create a new organisational structure or process to achieve this goal, separate from their own organisations;
- plan and implement a jointly agreed programme, often with joint staff or resources;
- share relevant information; and
- pool risks and rewards.

Glendinning et al (2005a, p 370) portray partnership working as follows:

> partnerships are defined as involving two or more organisations, groups or agencies that together identify, acknowledge and act to secure one or more common objective, interest or area of inter-dependence; but where the autonomy and separate accountability arrangements of the partner organisations are in principle retained.

Dickinson and Glasby (2010, p 815) use the same framework as Sullivan and Skelcher (2002), in which partnership:

> [involves] negotiation between people from different agencies committed to working together over more than the short term; aims to secure the delivery of benefits or added value which could not have been provided by any single agency acting alone or through the employment of others; and includes a formal articulation of a purpose and a plan to bind partners together.

However, one definition of collaboration by the Organisation for Economic Co-operation and Development (1990, p 18) is particularly appropriate in the context of our study of partnerships:

> Systems of formalised co-operation, grounded in legally binding arrangements or informal understandings, co-operative working relationships, and mutually adopted plans among a number of institutions. They involve agreements on policy and programme objectives and the sharing of

responsibility, resources, risks and benefits over a specified period of time.

It must be noted, however, that all these definitions have one feature in common: they do not prescribe areas, scope, structures or rationales for joint working (Glendinning et al, 2005a). These issues are addressed in the remainder of this chapter.

Why collaborate?

For the Audit Commission (1998, p 9), there are five main reasons why agencies develop partnerships:

• to deliver coordinated packages of services to individuals;
• to tackle so-called 'wicked issues';
• to reduce the impact of organisational fragmentation and minimise the impact of any perverse incentives that result from it;
• to bid for, or gain access to, new resources; and
• to meet a statutory requirement.

In a literature review of how to create successful partnerships, Wildridge et al (2004) argue that factors such as rapid change, decreased resources from government and the blurring of boundaries between the government, the public sector and voluntary and private sector organisations may facilitate the need for collaborative working. Huxham et al (2000) cite the need for increased efficiency as a main driver to work in partnership, inasmuch as organisations can create 'one-stop shops' for service users in order to create a seamless service. This also has the added advantages of shared learning between organisations and the opportunity to learn from best practice.

Dickinson and Glasby (2010, pp 820–1) conclude that: 'An extensive review of the network literature suggests that the majority [of networks] are driven by the need to secure access to resources, be they financial, workforce, knowledge, legitimacy and so on'. Glasby and Dickinson (2008, p 16) argue that the emphasis on a partnership approach could be attributed to a combination of the following factors:

• the increased fragmentation of services following the implementation of various market-based approaches to public services;
• the emphasis placed on 'customer satisfaction' by current political philosophies;

- the growth of various civil rights movements (around 'race', gender and disability), with service user-led organisations increasingly calling for services that enable them to lead chosen lifestyles (and for services that fit their lives, not the other way round);
- demographic changes (with older, more diverse and more mobile populations) and advances in medicine and technology leading to a need to deliver services in new and more cost-effective ways; and
- rising public expectations and a growing challenge to traditional professional power.

Arguably, one of the greatest drivers to work in partnership is the statutory obligation from central government. We discuss this topic in greater detail later in the chapter in relation to models and frameworks of partnership working. Once separate agencies, either through compulsion or collaborative advantage, have decided to work together, there are then a range of factors to consider, such as deciding: which partners to invite (or have to be included by statute); who to exclude; and what form and structures the partnership should take. As Powell and Dowling (2006) note, although there is very little theoretical literature on partnerships, there is no shortage of 'how to' guides on the subject (see, eg, the partnership assessment tool devised by Hardy et al [2003]). We now turn to look at some of the key elements that should be considered if collaborative agencies are to engage in a 'successful' partnership.

What makes for a 'successful' partnership?

Partnerships have the potential to make the delivery of services more seamless and coherent and therefore more efficient and effective. If each partner stands to gain in some manner from what they and other partners bring to the table in terms of additional resources and the pooling of ideas and knowledge, then it could be argued that partnerships bring value for each participant. These factors can generate new insights and ways to tackle problems and therefore partnerships can be more than the sum of their parts and bring a real synergy to tackling 'wicked issues' (Balloch and Taylor, 2001b). A number of policy guides and much of the academic literature have focused on what constitutes a 'successful' partnership. One must bear in mind that 'success' is a contested concept and what works for one partnership may not necessarily be the case for another. Policy and context matter greatly (Glasby and Dickinson, 2008; Williams and Sullivan, 2010).

In their review of the literature on how to create successful partnerships, Wildridge et al (2004) highlight a number of features:

- a common vision is key;
- trust is very important – sharing knowledge engenders trust;
- ensuring that smaller partners are seen as bringing equal value through their local knowledge and local legitimacy;
- clear consistent communication and including the views of service users;
- good decision-making and ensuring accountability with joint ownership of decisions adds collective accountability;
- a focus on outcomes; and
- people in place who can manage change.

In their systematic literature review highlighting the factors promoting and hindering joint working in health and social care, Cameron and Lart (2003) stress the following factors:

- strategic support and commitment;
- good communication;
- resources and personnel;
- strong management with appropriate professional support;
- past history of joint working;
- avoiding negative assessments and professional stereotypes;
- trust and respect; and
- joint training and team-building.

Cameron and Lart (2003) also highlight that joint aims and objectives that are understood by all partners are very important, as is ensuring that they are achievable. Clear roles and responsibilities between partners are also seen as key, with formal policy and procedures to ensure accountability and prevent duplication or gaps in provision.

The Partnership Assessment Tool (Hardy et al, 2003, p 14) identifies six partnership principles in creating a successful partnership:

- Principle 1 – Recognise and Accept the Need for Partnership.
- Principle 2 – Develop Clarity and Realism of Purpose.
- Principle 3 – Ensure Commitment and Ownership.
- Principle 4 – Develop and Maintain Trust.
- Principle 5 – Create Clear and Robust Partnership Arrangements.
- Principle 6 – Monitor, Measure and Learn.

The Audit Commission (1998, p 49), in their policy document *A fruitful partnership*, argue that the key ingredients for a successful partnership are:

- clear, shared objectives;
- a realistic plan and timetable for reaching these objectives;
- commitment from the partners to take the partnership's work into account within their mainstream activities;
- a clear framework of responsibilities and accountability;
- a high level of trust between partners; and
- realistic ways of measuring the partnership's achievements.

Cropper (cited in Hudson et al, 1999, p 247) sees organisations having a shared vision at the outset as important, and explicit statements of purpose are important because they:

- are a source of identity for collaborating organisations;
- help to clarify boundaries and commitments;
- define the scale and scope of joint work;
- serve as a way of raising and evaluating claims to membership of the collaborative;
- provide a control against collaborative drift; and
- provide a mechanism for the regulation of collaborative arrangements.

Powell et al (2001a) identify three elements making for a successful partnership. These manifest themselves through three streams: the policy stream, the process stream and the resource stream:

- *The policy stream* – are goals shared; are values shared and a consensus around ends and means recognised? Is there a shared vision of goals, priorities and objectives and the ordering of priorities?
- *The process stream* – highlights that the mechanism to achieve goals is comprised of three elements: instruments, ownership and jointness.
- *The resource stream* – human/financial resources, trust, information and the need for 'local champions' to drive the partnership agenda forward.

Finally, Hudson et al (1999, p 238) identify the 10 components of collaborative endeavour:

1. Contextual factors: expectations and constraints.
2. Recognition of the need to collaborate.
3. Identification of a legitimate basis for collaboration.

4. Assessment of collaborative capacity.
5. Articulation of a clear sense of collaborative purpose.
6. Building up trust from principled conduct.
7. Ensuring wide organisational ownership.
8. Nurturing fragile relationships.
9. Selection of an appropriate collaborative relationship.
10. Selection of a pathway.

What these examples from the literature tell us is that having a common vision among partners is of great importance to ensure that they are all clear about the aims and objectives of the partnership and what it is there to achieve. Trust is paramount to effective partnership working: it is the 'glue' that not only holds the partnership together, but sustains and nurtures it. The partnership has to be clear that its goals are achievable and not set so high as to become some abstract 'mission statement' that is vague, unworkable and doomed to failure. Conversely, if expectations are set too low, this may mean that only peripheral issues are addressed and there is a danger that partners may lose interest (Ranade and Hudson, 2003). Systematic and regular monitoring is required to ensure that the partnership is on track, and effective and committed collaborative leadership at a senior level is essential.

Of course, how these various factors get played out in actual practice, their respective weighting and the balance between them will vary according to the particular partnership in question, its purpose and the context in which it is located. Beyond a certain level, generalising about the ingredients of a successful partnership may not be especially helpful. As Balloch and Taylor (2001b, p 7) argue: 'there can be no blueprint for successful partnerships. Rather, each partnership needs to find a balance between the flexibility that partnerships require if they are to break new ground. Finding that balance requires skills that are not always available'.

Moreover, having clearly specified goals may not in fact be possible in an area of considerable uncertainty, like public health, where specifying the goal in advance may either not be possible or could possibly be misleading and perhaps result in unintended consequences. Rather, the goal may be emergent and become evident only once those engaged in finding solutions to the problem start to tackle it. As Huxham (2003, p 404, emphasis in original) observes:

> It appears to be *common wisdom* that it is necessary to be clear about the aims of joint working if partners are to work together to operationalize policies. Typically people argue

for common (or at least compatible), agreed or clear sets of aims as a starting point in collaboration. The *common practice*, however, appears to be that the variety of organizational and individual agendas that are present in collaborative situations make it difficult to agree on aims in practice.

Although Cropper (cited in Hudson et al, 1999) gave us reasons for having a shared vision, there is also the caveat that there is a danger of being too prescriptive and that partnerships should be allowed to develop their own themes and strategies. However, rather than accept, or even embrace, the unavoidable messiness of public health issues, the instinctive reaction is usually to reduce complexity and try to achieve greater certainty in order to move into the simple system zone (Chapman, 2004). So, if a partnership is seen not to be working, the temptation is to resort to a reductionist or essentially mechanistic approach by proposing that the partnership be made statutory, or by strengthening monitoring arrangements to ensure that the partnership delivers what it promises or has been set up to achieve. We return to these issues later in the chapter in relation to 'mandatory partnerships' and systems thinking.

Models and frameworks of partnership working

As McDonald (2005, p 579) notes:

> At the level of theory, partnership working has been presented as a critique of both market- and state-led forms of governance, while in policy discourse it is presented as offering the potential for a more resource efficient, outcome-effective and inclusive-progressive form of policy delivery.

To understand partnerships, we have to understand the models, frameworks and contexts in which they operate. Partnerships do not operate in a policy vacuum and contextual factors such as legislation, policy directives, targets, political ideology and so on will shape the form and function of the partnerships and their *modus operandi*. Glasby and Dickinson (2008), among others (see, eg, Lowndes and Skelcher, 1998; Hudson et al, 1999; Ranade and Hudson, 2003), argue that partnerships should be seen in the context of hierarchies, markets and networks.

As Ranade and Hudson (2003, p 34) note:

> Social science literature identifies three 'pure' routes to social co-ordination or governance – hierarchy, markets and networks ... and these provide a useful starting point for analysing the recent history of public service delivery and hence the context within which current collaborations take place.

Glasby and Dickinson (2008) observe that partnerships can intersect with all three modes of governance. They see the three strands as follows:

- *Hierarchy* – often a single organisation with 'top-down' rules and procedures, and with statutes governing how the organisation works.
- *Market* – multiple organisations competitively trading goods and services on price.
- *Network* – seen as lying between a hierarchy and a market, with multiple organisations coming together informally, based on shared outlook or priorities or interpersonal relationships.

A hierarchy is characterised by rules of governance; a market is driven by incentives; and interactions are the quintessence of networks. Lowndes and Skelcher's (1998) table highlights the features of all three models (see Table 2.1).

Table 2.1: Mode of governance – market, hierarchy and network

	Market	Hierarchy	Network
Normative basis	Contract – property rights	Employment relationship	Complementary strengths
Means of communication	Prices	Routines	Relational
Methods of conflict resolution	Haggling – resort to courts	Administrative fiat – supervision	Norm of reciprocity – reputational concerns
Degree of flexibility	High	Low	Medium
Amount of commitment among the parties	Low	Medium	High
Tone or climate	Precision and/or suspicion	Formal, bureaucratic	Open-ended, mutual benefits
Actor preferences or choices	Independent	Dependent	Interdependent

Source: Lowndes and Skelcher (1998, p 319); adapted from Powell (1991, p 269).

Lowndes and Skelcher (1998) argue that a *market* mode of governance revolves around contractual relationships over property rights, and price mechanisms are the way transactions are conducted. In the event of a dispute, haggling or recourse to the law are the means to resolve such issues. It is argued that markets provide a high degree of flexibility to actors in forming alliances, although given the competitive nature of a market, suspicion may underline any collaborative undertaking. Collaboration in a market environment will be largely opportunistic to gain competitive advantage.

Theoretically, Lowndes and Skelcher (1998) argue that the *hierarchical* mode of governance overcomes the difficulties of participation in competitive markets. With an authoritative integrating and supervisory structure, this enables bureaucratic routines to be established. Coordination of roles is undertaken by administrative 'command-and-control' mechanisms. The downside of such mechanisms is that there is a reduction in flexibility and a lack of innovation because of a tendency to formalisation of roles and responsibilities and their routine nature.

Finally, the *network* mode of governance sees actors as being able to identify corresponding interests. The development of collaborative relationships based on loyalty, trust and reciprocity allows mutual action to occur. With their voluntary nature, Lowndes and Skelcher (1998) argue that networks establish and maintain the allegiance of members over the longer term. Disputes are determined in a network approach on the basis of members' reputational concerns.

Partnerships, it is argued, fluctuate between all three modes of governance according to the life cycle of the partnership. In a pre-partnership collaboration, the relationships between partners will be informal, with some element of trust and cooperation. There is a need to work together because, for example, of similar interests or goals, in addition to the recognition that each partner has access to crucial but different resources. This then could well describe a network mode of governance, with informality and trust being prominent. As the partnership negotiates over membership and policy and procedures are drawn up and roles allocated and codified, the former informal arrangements are replaced by formal hierarchical structures and decision making procedures, with a partnership board, for example, being established.

As the partnership moves on to delivering its formalised plans of delivery, Lowndes and Skelcher (1998) argue that it then moves into a market mode of governance. Tendering, contracting out and service level agreements with various service providers (who may or may not be part of the partnership) accentuate this stage of the life cycle of the partnership, with monitoring and regulating of the contractors. The market approach is characterised by low levels of cooperation between providers and purchasers and distinctions may arise between those who have contracts or service level agreements and those who do not, resulting in insider/outsider status of the partnership.

Finally, at the partnership termination and succession phase, there is uncertainty among partners as the collaboration comes to an end, but with this comes the potential for openness and further collaboration among some partners, with trust again coming to the fore, and perhaps a need to maintain community involvement or retain staff. This loosening of formal relations is indicative of a network mode of governance (Lowndes and Skelcher, 1998). With the fluctuation between all three modes of governance, Lowndes and Skelcher (1998) argue that partnerships are therefore not purely based upon mutual benefit, trust and reciprocity, all characteristics of a network approach.

Ranade and Hudson (2003, p 36), discussing networks in the context of the three modes of governance, argue that:

> The key feature of the network mode of governance is that co-ordination is achieved by less formal and more egalitarian means than the other two models, and explicit attention is paid to the way co-operation and trust are formed and maintained ... the 'entangling strings' of reputation, friendship, interdependence and altruism all become an integral part of the relationship, and that the information obtained is thereby both 'thicker' than that in the market and 'freer' than that communicated in a hierarchy.

They also concur with Lowndes and Skelcher (1998) that partnerships operate in and *overlay* a complex, fluid and dynamic policy governance framework of hierarchy, market and network in a variety of settings. In this way, partnerships operate in a hybrid model of governance, which Ranade and Hudson (2003) argue is in part due to New Labour promoting partnerships while simultaneously giving a greater role to the voluntary, community and private sectors in bidding to run services, as well as to the greater focus on initiatives such as the Private Finance Initiative, combined with a target and performance management culture.

Powell and Dowling (2006), in comparing conceptual models of partnership, cite Stoker's model, which emphasises three types of partnership:

- *Principal–agent partnerships* involve purchaser–provider relationships, such as the contracts associated with competitive tendering and 'best value'.
- *Inter-organisational negotiation* involves bargaining and coordination between parties through the blending of capacities (such as in Single Regeneration Budget partnerships).
- *Systemic coordination* goes further by establishing a level of being embedded and of mutual understanding to the extent that organisations develop a shared vision and degree of joint working, which leads to the establishment of self-governing networks.

Arguably, all three frameworks bear more than a passing resemblance to the market, hierarchy and network modes of governance. The 'Principal–agent partnerships', with their emphasis on contractual relations and competitive tendering, share many similarities with the market mode of governance. The 'Inter-organisational negotiation' model would appear to fit the hierarchical mode of governance, with its emphasis upon bargaining and coordinating between parties and the agency at the centre coordinating bureaucratic relations and creating frameworks and structures. Stoker's 'Systemic coordination' model fits with the ethos of the network mode of governance, with its emphasis on mutual understanding, shared vision and, as Stoker points out, the establishment of self-governing networks.

When we look at how partnerships may operate within these frameworks in the policy and contextual context, it is helpful to refer to Hudson's 'framework for collaboration', which forms a continuum from Isolation, through Encounter, Communication and Collaboration, to Integration (cited in Powell et al, 2001):

- Isolation – no joint activity.
- Encounter – some contact but informal, ad hoc and marginal to the goals of the organisations.
- Communication – organisations joint working within a formal and structured nature, but which tends to be separate and marginal to an organisation's own goals.
- Collaboration – recognition by organisations that partnership working is central to their mainstream activities, implying a trusting relationship, with organisations seeing each other as reliable partners.
- Integration – collaboration so high that organisations see their separate identities as insignificant.

As we have seen, partnerships may fluctuate between these activities depending on the mode of governance (hierarchy, market or network), and may exhibit some of these features simultaneously. For example, in a contractual dispute, there may be little or no contact between partners, or where partners are engaged in a policy network, there may be such a high level of integration (eg between two voluntary organisations offering similar services) that it is both practical and desirable for an integrated approach. Rhodes (cited in Hudson et al, 1999) argues that policy networks may display a continuum from high integration, in which policy communities are tightly integrated in the policymaking process and are characterised by a stable but restrictive membership, to the other end of the continuum populated by what is termed 'issue' networks, which are looser, with less stable membership and weak points of entry. Balloch and Taylor (2001a) believe that partnership working can be divided into four types of behaviour – competition, cooperation, coordination and co-evolution – with true partnerships having elements of each and the possibility of movement between them. Wildridge et al (2004) cite Gray (1989), who distinguishes between collaboration (a temporary and evolving forum for addressing a problem), cooperation (informal arrangements to achieve reciprocity) and coordination (formal institutional relationships). Gray notes that collaboration can entail cooperation and coordination, much the same as partnerships can display elements of hierarchy and network, for example.

Snape and Stewart (cited in Powell et al, 2006, p 306) identify three types of partnership: facilitating, coordinating and implementing:

- *Facilitating partnerships* manage entrenched, highly problematic, contentious or politically sensitive issues in which issues of power are at stake, with trust and solidarity being essential for success.
- *Coordinating partnerships* focus on less contentious issues where partners agree on priorities but are equally concerned with other pressing demands specific to themselves.
- *Implementing partnerships* are more pragmatic and time limited, concerned with specific and mutually beneficial projects.

Snape and Stewart's framework is especially useful as it adds the dimension of policy context, in addition to the environment in which partners operate (eg network, hierarchy, market).

Finally, Glasby and Dickinson (2008) posit that there are optimist, pessimist and realist approaches to partnership working. These are outlined in Table 2.2.

It could be argued that the characteristics of the optimist, pessimist and realist approaches share many similarities with the network, market and hierarchy modes of governance. Like the network approach, optimists believe in coming together because they have a shared vision and interests and they view their potential partners in optimistic terms, with high levels of trust and a belief in collaboration for its own sake. Boundary spanners and 'local champions' characterise the network approach, especially at the front-line level, as we will show in Chapter Five. Pessimists could be said in many circumstances to equate with the market approach, with a belief in maintaining or enhancing an organisation's position — it is characterised by a rather individualistic approach, as opposed to the altruistic network approach. The view of other partners reflects their own motivations, which is that the partnership essentially exists for one's own gain. The key reason for working in partnership is to ensure one's own survival — a 'survival of the fittest', 'dog eat dog' mentality that arguably coincides with a pure market-oriented approach. Finally, the realist approach could be said to resemble in many respects the hierarchy approach, in that the realist, like the bureaucratic hierarchy, is responding to events and not initiating them, and the 'rules of the game' have already been made. The realisation is that change is needed because other organisations have come to this conclusion and therefore it had better 'get with the programme'. It needs to do this because of a realisation that it will otherwise be left behind — in other words, 'adapt or die' or, rather more prosaically, be left

Table 2.2: Optimist, pessimist and realist approaches to partnership working

	Optimist	Pessimist	Realist
Why collaboration happens?	Achieving shared vision	Maintaining/ enhancing position	Responding to new environments
Key assumptions about other partners	Altruistic	Seeking personal or organisational gain	Realise need to change as society changes
Key factors at work	Role of charismatic leaders/boundary spanners	Power of individual partners and desire for survival	Ability to adapt to changing environment

Source: Glasby and Dickinson (2008, p 80); adapted from Sullivan and Skelcher (2002).

out of the loop. Of course, in New Labour's conception of partnerships, this is not entirely true, due to the mandatory element requiring many organisations to work in partnership, which does question many of the assumptions about the nature of partnership working, a matter to which we now turn.

When is a partnership not a partnership?

Mandatory partnerships may seem something of an oxymoron, but with the election of New Labour, they were an oxymoron made statute. As the Audit Commission (1998, p 5) highlighted a year after the election of the first New Labour administration: 'Mandatory partnership working is set to expand significantly as the Government implements its commitments to partnerships covering crime and disorder, health action zones, health improvement plans, youth offending teams, education action zones and early years development plans'. Within a few years, mandatory partnership working became a key feature, particularly in the public health arena. We explore this in more detail in Chapter Three through a focus on a systematic literature review of public health partnerships under New Labour conducted as part of the research reported in Chapters Four and Five.

Hudson (2004, p 76, emphasis in original) argues that: 'in a range of different policy areas, a stream of legislation, guidance and regulation has been directed towards the idea that the centre can *compel* the creation of partnerships at local level – the creation of partnership by hierarchy'. He goes on to argue that this 'top-down' hierarchical approach may work for partnerships where the goals are clear and the strategy is known on how to achieve such goals, but where collective goals are less clear and the time frame is long, and the strategy required to achieve such goals is unclear, then such an approach may not be suitable.

Clarke and Glendinning (2002, p 46, emphasis in original) argue that:

> New Labour's compulsory partnerships ... [are] an attempt to recruit *subordinated* partners into the project of 'modernising' government. Such subordinate roles certainly allow some autonomy and initiative in the process of working together. However, this autonomy is bounded; it's circumscribed by central direction and resource control; is subject to surveillance and evaluation; and is vulnerable to termination or takeover.

Because of this 'statutory voluntarism', many partnerships, particularly public health partnerships, are differentiated from a network governance approach by virtue of a partnership board not being made up of willing partners, but of agencies there under duress in a 'shotgun marriage'. Therefore, relations are not built upon trust, mutual benefit and reciprocity – characteristics that are the hallmarks of network governance. Partnerships in this sense resemble a quasi-network, that is, an intermediate form of organisation not quite conforming to a hierarchy or market model (Powell and Exworthy, 2002). Dickinson and Glasby (2010) argue that not all partnerships can be equated to networks and a number of partnerships may appear more akin to hierarchies (eg Care Trusts) or market-based relationships (eg public–private partnerships) than to horizontal and trust-based ones, as networks tend to be characterised.

As we have seen, partnerships can be partly based on altruism, but also on self-interest. Mackintosh (1993) distinguishes between three types of partnership according to what partners want out of it: a budget enlargement partnership; a 'synergy' or 'added value' partnership; and a 'transformation' model of partnership. The budget enlargement model is used to combine resources. The 'synergy' or 'added value' model is aimed at increasing value by combining assets and powers of separate organisations, and the aim of the 'transformation' model emphasises changes in the aims and cultures of partner organisations. This depends upon the power of partner organisations. For instance, where organisations have roughly equal power, there may be bilateral changes, and where one organisation has more power, there may in effect be a takeover, isomorphism or virtual integration by the more powerful organisation. The 'transformation' model is where agencies have a different focus and priorities.

With these models partners may have different relationships depending on the extent to which partnerships are based on hierarchical, market or network principles, in addition to the existence of different partnership cultures (Balloch and Taylor, 2001a). However, as Ranade and Hudson (2003, p 48) note: 'The rhetoric which currently surrounds inter-organisational collaboration as an attractive ideal cloaks the fact that the network mode of social organisation coexists with, and is embedded in, other modes based on hierarchies and markets'.

Rummery (2002, p 243), in evaluating New Labour's approach to partnerships, concludes that: 'partnerships New Labour-style appear to embrace a mixture of quasi-market style incentives with bureaucratic, statist controls; only in some, rare, cases does the state adopt a laissez-faire enabling approach that might signify a true commitment to a "Third Way" networked governance'.

Barriers to partnership working

Cameron and Lart (2003, p 9) note that:

> The problems associated with joint working and joint planning have long been recognised. Studies of the then newly created Joint Consultative Committees and Joint Planning structures, published in the 1980s, identified differences in professional cultures, organisational structures and forms of accountability.

As illustrated earlier, partnership working is hardly a new phenomenon and neither are the problems associated with it, which are many and varied. As Glasby and Dickinson, 2008, p xvi) argue: 'In practice, anyone who has ... worked in health and social care knows that partnership working can be both frustrating and messy – even if you follow the so-called "rules"'. The Audit Commission (1998, p 7) highlights the following barriers to working in partnership:

- getting partners to agree on priorities for action;
- keeping partners actively involved;
- preventing the partnership from becoming simply a talking shop;
- making decisions that all partners endorse;
- deciding who will provide the resources needed to achieve the partnership's objectives;
- linking the partnership's work with partners' mainstream activities and budgets;
- monitoring the partnership's effectiveness;
- working out whether what is achieved justifies the costs involved; and
- avoiding 'partnership overload', particularly where agencies are each involved in large numbers of partnerships.

They also note that partnership working is often expensive, as well as difficult. Many of the costs involved are not recorded and few partnerships have precise information about them.

The World Health Organization (2012, p 59), in its literature review of why collaborative governance can fail, found:

- conflict about goals and objectives;

- considerable but underestimated direct and opportunity costs in terms of the time it takes to build trust and consensus;
- weak accountability of partners for success or failure;
- territorial and organisational difficulties when partnerships are seen as detracting from existing mainstream initiatives or when features of the structures or institutions within the partnering agencies make it particularly difficult to break out of policy silos;
- asymmetrical technical skills and expertise for contributing to the partnership;
- differences in philosophy among partners, such as the role of markets, or different value or ethical systems, which fragment the partnership's cooperative culture; and
- differing power relations and levels of community participation.

These are all compelling difficulties for creating effective collaborative advantage, but Williams and Sullivan (2010, p 10) make an important point, and one that is rarely encountered in the literature on partnerships, which may have a bearing on some of the previous points: 'It is somewhat perverse that we countenance "unskilled" people working in collaborative settings when we would never entertain such a situation in the management of individual public services'. They go on to highlight that training and development budgets are currently directed to mainstream professional and managerial development but not to how to work collaboratively. Perhaps some of the problems of joint working are that we just throw individuals and organisations in 'at the deep end' and it is literally 'sink or swim' as they do not have the skills or competencies to work in partnership, having never done so before; further, this is without all the structural, administrative and cultural barriers highlighted earlier that have to be negotiated. Research by Penhale et al (2007) on partnership working in safeguarding vulnerable adults found that social care staff and partner agencies working on the front line would have valued more collaborative training, or any training, in order to learn how other agencies contributed to working in partnership to protect some of the most vulnerable in society. It is this gap in leadership and management development that led to the design of a programme that is based explicitly on whole-systems thinking rooted in improvement science and partnership working (Hannaway et al, 2007; Hunter, 2007a). It would seem that the absence of such training and development is more evident in public health settings than in others that focus, in particular, on health care services.

Other factors can create barriers to partnership working that are beyond the control of an individual, such as ideological differences, a history of antagonism, professional tribalism and a lack of resources to service the partnership (Wildridge et al, 2004). Hardy (cited in Powell and Exworthy, 2001) highlights five categories of barriers to collaboration in regard to social care: structural, procedural, financial, professional and status legitimacy. These categories arguably also hold true for partnership working in general, including partnerships in public health. They are certainly evident in public health in England given the evolution of the speciality and the power struggles between those who are medically qualified and those who are not, as described in Chapter One.

As noted, the time, energy and commitment required by individuals and organisations is also a major obstacle to effective partnership working. Williams and Sullivan (2010, p 7), in their study of partnerships, found this to be the case and report that:

> There was a sense that, although the rhetoric of collaboration was strong, the default position of many organisations was self-interest and turf protection, and that collaboration was often perceived as an additional responsibility and a call on limited resources and time, not an integral part of an organisation's core business.

Other studies have found that there is a tendency for agencies to burden staff who already have heavy workloads with the additional responsibilities of partnership working and rely on their goodwill to ensure that any collaborative endeavours are a success (see, eg, Hills et al, 2007; Dickinson, 2008; Williams and Sullivan, 2010).

Hudson et al (1999) point to two significant barriers to working in partnership: first, that an individual agency may lose some of its autonomy and freedom to act independently and as such may prefer to keep control over its own affairs rather than invest time and resources in the partnership when the returns are far from clear and possibly intangible; and, second, that just as partnership working can bring success, the potential downside for some agencies may be that they do not bask in the glory all on their own but have to share the credit with another organisation or even let it take the full credit for a successful endeavour. The tensions here are between retaining organisational flexibility and control on the one hand, and the construction of joint agendas that might mean surrendering some power and control on the other. At the same time, organisations may also face pressures to tighten control and become more focused and less flexible depending upon their size, structure and status.

Furthermore, power and control also mean certain partner organisations can control access to the partnership and, as alluded to earlier, this can lead to an insider/outsider status for certain partners. At best, some partners may be nothing more than peripheral members. This is true for smaller members, such as those from the third sector, and as Ranade and Hudson (2003, p 42) explain: 'Poorly resourced or marginalised groups find it difficult to "break in" to the networks, or get access to relevant, timely information, leading to suspicions that partnership decisions are "sewn up" in advance between the insiders'. This concern is also made by Balloch and Taylor (2001a), who argue that smaller partners from the third sector do not have the resources to engage effectively in partnerships.

Barriers to working in partnership can also occur through national policy, such as directives to deliver on targets, organisational change, new policy frameworks, tensions in power relations and so on. It is to these matters that we now turn.

Delivering through partnerships

Even if perfect conditions are present, and no barriers are in place to scupper progress, a major problem with partnerships is not knowing, or not being certain, that any achievements that occur can be tracked back to the partnership. There will be those who stand by their partnerships as having been effective but they will be hard-pressed to provide tangible evidence. As Pollitt (2003, p 61) points out: 'academic research does not indicate that the partnership form [or forms] ... regularly produce[s] performance gains. In other words, we cannot assume that they usually "work", in terms of delivering better programmes'. Huxham and Vangen (2000) found from their research that those involved in partnerships often commented that 'little is being achieved'. They conclude that 'it is not uncommon for people to argue that positive outputs have happened despite the partnership rather than because of it' (Huxham and Vangen, 2000, p 294).

Partnerships: policy, practice and context

How partnerships respond to policy challenges, particularly around 'wicked issues', is in large part based upon the structural context, that is, the political, policy and cultural environments in which partnerships operate and to what extent such factors can shape not only partnerships, but also their response to policy problems. As Huxham et al (2000, p 346) note: 'Structural issues are important because they affect the way collaborative agendas are formed and implemented'. Structural issues play an important role because they shape the policy environment and dictate the way partnerships can or cannot respond to the policy agenda in regard to the capacity to act, the resources available and the access to, and influence on, policy levers based upon status and power.

Partnerships and power

Government policy and the power relationship between central and local government can have a major impact on the effectiveness of partnerships in a number of ways, including the following:

- imposing conflicting high-level objectives. These objectives may include a target that is a high priority for central government but is not an issue at local level; for example, a government target to decrease teenage pregnancy by a certain percentage in a local authority where teenage pregnancy rates are already very low would not be a priority for the local authority. Government targets can also mean that agencies concentrate on their own government-imposed targets and not the priorities of the partnership (Huxham et al, 2000);

- restricting agencies' ability to pool resources and information. Many studies have discussed how such matters as data protection or lack of information-sharing protocols have prevented partner agencies sharing information (see Speller, 1999; Benzeval and Meth, 2002; CRESR, 2005; Freeman and Peck, 2006), and even with the Health Act 1999, which introduced health flexibilities (allowing organisations to pool budgets), there are still a number of problems around resources and pooling budgets (see Arora et al, 1999, 2000; Bauld et al, 2001; Powell et al, 2001; Matka et al, 2002; Sullivan et al, 2002; Benzeval, 2003; Mackenzie et al, 2003; Hills et al, 2007);

- changes in government policy that render some priorities of the partnership less important or redundant;

- limiting or diluting the powers available to agencies to address problems through agreements on funding arrangements or restrictions on the use of resources, financial services or sanctions (Glendinning et al, 2005b), which in turn distort locally identified needs and priorities;

- partnerships being reluctant to undertake government priorities that interfere with the local implementation of present programmes and, more importantly, dilute local ownership of the partnership, which may result in agencies leaving the partnership as they see their priorities and goals subordinated by government priorities (Hudson, 2004); and

- mandatory partnerships in which certain partners are deemed by the government as ex officio automatically creating insider/outsider status (Audit Commission, 1998).

Power relationships at a local level also have an impact on the ability of partnerships to respond to the policy problems that they were created to solve. Imbalances in local power relationships can mean that certain partners dominate the policy agenda and processes and certain priorities are either left off the agenda or are not even considered to be worth putting on in the first place. This means that less powerful partners and the concerns of their constituent members are effectively sidelined and the agenda is monopolised by professional providers, with the less powerful partners excluded from decisions around, for example, strategic planning and service delivery (Balloch and Taylor, 2001a). Of course, which partners have the most power is largely dictated by central government, as Rummery (2002, p 243) notes: 'Partnership working New Labour-style benefits powerful partners'. Huxham (2003) argues that those who have the ability to invite members onto the partnership and to allot to which section of the partnership agencies are assigned have power.

Powell and Exworthy (2002, p 26) pose an interesting question in this regard: '[if] power asymmetries set a limit to networks how much inequality of power is possible before a network becomes a hierarchy?' This has particular resonance with the inclusion of government targets and priorities. McDonald (2005) goes further and argues that partnerships are nothing more than a mechanism for nullifying dissent thorough incorporation and are used by elites to keep power and reinforce existing power relations. Partnerships do little to empower users and divert resources away from welfare delivery. Lowndes and Skelcher (1998, p 331) believe that: 'What remains unanswered – and, to some extent, unasked – are the conventional questions of the pluralist debate: who has power, who gains and who loses as the policy makers' obsession with networks and partnerships grows?' Powell et al (2001, p 59) provide the following answer: 'the rules of the game are laid down by the centre'.

Speaking a different language? Cultural barriers and partnerships

Members of partnerships bring their own values, beliefs and behaviours, which could be loosely termed 'corporate culture', which can have a bearing on partnerships and power relationships. Ranade and Hudson (2003) argue that cultural norms and behaviour can impact on partnerships in terms of importing hierarchies of power, resources, status and styles of leadership – these may be facilitative or 'top-down', depending on the organisation. Balloch and Taylor (2001a) argue that each organisation may be set in its ways and a lot of professional resistance and cultural expectations need to be overcome in partnership working. These cultural differences can lead to cultural stereotyping between professionals and result in a lack of agreement about roles, responsibilities and other issues. Hudson et al (1999, p 246, emphasis in original) argue that: 'any interpretation of organizational culture must be deeply embedded in the contextual richness of the total social life of organizational members – culture is something that the organization *is*, rather than a variable that can be manipulated by management'. Therefore, organisational culture is not something that can be performance managed or modified by central diktat. Changing cultural beliefs and expectations in a partnership will take time and may only ever be partially successful. Cultural differences can also lead to misunderstandings, for example, someone from a local authority may view health inequalities from a social model of health whereas an NHS representative may think more in terms of a medical model of health. In addition, representatives may not understand each other's organisational jargon and certain groups, particularly those from the voluntary and community sector, may feel excluded (Huxham et al, 2000).

Time for a new approach?

As we have sought to show, in order to create a successful partnership, certain key decisions need to be made at the outset and stated in a plan that has the agreement of all potential partners. These decisions include:

- clarifying and agreeing lines of responsibility;
- identifying and stating achievable goals;
- systematic and regular monitoring to ensure that the partnership is on track;
- effective and committed collaborative leadership at a senior level; and

- ensuring trust, which is an important ingredient among those taking part in partnerships.

As discussed earlier, how these various factors get enacted, their respective weighting and the balance between them will vary according to each partnership, its rationale and the context in which it is located. As we have seen, partnerships, particularly public health partnerships, face many challenges and have to address a myriad of 'wicked issues', but rather than explore adaptive systems and different nuanced approaches to tackling such 'wicked issues', the instinctive reaction is usually to try to reduce complexity and simplify systems (Chapman, 2004).

Such tinkering with existing arrangements and constructs may provide temporary or minimal relief, but it will more likely disappoint. In contrast to rational, linear and reductionist thinking, as noted earlier, systems thinking posits that it is better to try multiple approaches and let the desired direction arise by focusing on those things that seem to be working best, that is, adopting an emergent approach. Seddon (2008, p 70) argues that it means thinking 'about the organisation from the outside-in' in order 'to integrate decision-making with work' – it is to understand the nature of the task or problem to be tackled and to design a system that meets it.

So, according to this way of viewing the world, new possibilities are explored through experimentation and through working at the edge of what is known. Getting heads around the problem is certainly desirable but perhaps not through pre-existing and often over-engineered partnerships that themselves may militate against finding new ways of tackling complex problems. A systems perspective challenges the accepted ways of managing and governing affairs, viewing them as part of the problem rather than the solution. Systems failure occurs when the capacity of a system to adapt is no longer possible. The consequence is a growing sense of distance, disillusion and frustration in those designing policy and those implementing it. A possible reason, then, for partnership underperformance or failure is the misplaced attention focused on structures and systems, which, perhaps unintentionally, has resulted in limiting the adaptive potential of partnerships that is essential for tackling 'wicked issues' (Chapman, 2004).

The notion of 'backward-mapping' is helpful in understanding this relationship between those designing and implementing policy, respectively (Elmore, 1979). For Elmore, the critical issues are where, in the complex welter of relationships at the delivery level, are the individuals who have the closest proximity to the problems, and what resources, financial and otherwise, do they have to address them? In

---

45

this sense, the goal of backward-mapping is to isolate the one or two critical points in a complex multi-partner relationship of the type under study in the research reported in later chapters that have the closest proximity to the problem, and identify what needs to happen at those points to solve the problem or meet the objective.

Systems thinking does not offer a panacea or a 'silver bullet' solution or magically make complex problems disappear (Chapman, 2004); it demonstrates that managing complex adaptive systems demands a new mindset that may be more focused on improving what can be done rather than trying to meet a specified target or goal that may be unrealistic, unattainable or just wrong. Adopting a systems perspective, the process of designing, formulating and implementing policies is based more on the facilitation of improvements than on control of the organisation or system. As Chapman (2004, p 87) puts it: 'the aim should be to provide a minimum specification that creates an environment in which innovative, complex behaviours can emerge'. Moreover, the leadership style within a systems approach will be based more on listening, asking questions and co-producing possible solutions than on telling and instructing. Reinforcing these insights are others from an Institute of Government study on how government can perform better. The researchers conclude:

> We try to avoid assuming that collaboration implies neat and tidy organisational structures and processes, or that it depends upon formal coordination machinery. Indeed, our research clearly shows that the real value of effective joining-up mechanisms lies in their ability to foster new kinds of conversations and relationships between key players in government. *These relationships cannot be over-engineered – effective problem-solving may sometimes come, at least in theory, from competition, conflict and even a little chaos at the margin.* (Parker et al, 2010, p 74, emphasis added)

A similar argument is put forward by Leadbeater (1999), who maintains that the problem of sclerosis in public services can be put down to public organisations having been designed as bureaucracies to process large numbers of cases in identical ways. A feature of such organisations is their division into 'professionally dominated departments with activity concentrated into narrow specialisms, with little cross-fertilisation of ideas or practices' (Leadbeater, 1999, p 206). Generally, as a consequence, public organisations 'have heavy-handed management systems which provide limited autonomy or personal responsibility for front-line staff'

(Leadbeater, 1999, p 206). Leadbeater accepts that trust is essential for effective partnership working but challenges the notion that it can only be present where long-term sustainable relationships have been nurtured and allowed to survive and flourish. He suggests that such an argument may be overstated and used to provide a convenient excuse for partnership failure. He believes that some of the most creative and productive relationships are often based on intense, short-term trust and points to the film, advertising and entertainment industries as being successful examples of such an approach. He cites the example of a film crew coming together to make a film. They may not know one another but will work intensely together over a few weeks or months to get the film made. In contrast, he argues that long-term trusting relationships, where they do still exist, risk becoming (if they are not already) cosy and collusive affairs that give rise to problems of their own that, paradoxically, can make long-term, mutual trust the enemy of creative and innovative joint working.

Partnerships could conceivably operate in a different manner, as suggested by the earlier examples, thereby providing an appropriate mechanism for applying a systems approach. However, from the available evidence, it does not seem that many, if any, partnerships in practice function in such a way and rarely, if ever, in public health hitherto. Like the host organisations that spawned them, and to which they report, they seem to be more comfortable operating in a reductionist mode rather than a systems mode. Part of the reason for this is the highly prescriptive context in which they have been set up and are managed – a notable feature of the public service reforms implemented in the period from around 2000 (Hunter, 2003, 2008b). Adopting a systems perspective requires being non-prescriptive about means, so that only a minimum specification is deemed necessary. This would then allow an opportunity to test out different partnership approaches and styles, rejecting those that were not successful while retaining those that seemed to work (see Table 2.3). This approach is in harmony with a pure network approach, rather than a hierarchical or market mode of governance.

As noted earlier, partnerships are a slippery topic (Pollitt, 2003). They may generally be deemed 'a good thing' in rhetorical terms, but whether they are in practice is dependent upon many factors that will be specific to the particular problem or issue that a partnership is set up to tackle. Conceivably, adopting a systems perspective may help overcome some of the problems and limitations associated with partnerships, and identified in the literature, so that they can become more effective. Building and managing partnerships is essential to a systems perspective, but different skills from those commonly found are needed to enable them to work effectively (Hunter, 2008a). The type of skills needed for systems thinking compared with more traditional, reductionist approaches are illustrated in Table 2.3.

Commonly identified problems with, and limitations of, partnerships are often the converse of the success factors described in this chapter, namely, poor or weak leadership, an absence of resources and incentives to facilitate effective partnerships, no clear or consistent goals, a lack of trust, and so on. There can also be problems over accountability, where no single partner feels fully accountable for the actions of the partnership. Invariably, responsibility is split across the partners, which can give rise to the question 'Who is in charge?'. The transaction costs involved in taking part in and servicing partnerships also need to be identified and accounted for since they can be significant. Unless they can be offset against clear benefits associated with partnerships, then it may be that their value can (and should) be challenged. Added to

Table 2.3: Skills of systems thinking

Usual approach	Systems thinking approach
Static thinking	*Dynamic thinking*
Focusing on particular events	Framing a problem in terms of a pattern of behaviour over time
Systems-as-effect thinking	*Systems-as-cause thinking*
Viewing behaviour generated by a system as driven by external forces	Placing responsibility for a behaviour on internal actors who manage the policies and 'plumbing' of the system
Tree-by-tree thinking	*Forest thinking*
Believing that really knowing something means focusing on the details	Believing that to know something requires understanding the context of relationships
Factors thinking	*Operational thinking*
Listing factors that influence or correlate with some result	Concentrating on causality and understanding how a behaviour is generated
Straight-line thinking	*Loop thinking*
Viewing causality as running in one direction, ignoring (either deliberately or not) the interdependence and interaction between and among the causes	Viewing causality as an ongoing process, not a one-time event, with effect feeding back to influence the causes and the causes affecting each other

Source: De Savigny and Adam (2009, p 43).

these potential problems are many others arising from organisational difficulties, including differences in missions and values, professional orientations, structures, and political settings (eg the NHS and local government, respectively). At a strategic level, and this point is highly pertinent to the study reported in this book, effective partnership working may be undermined by the rigidity of prevailing institutional and policy structures. As we noted earlier, such vertical 'silos' are a feature of the way government departments and agencies operate and are organised, but the effect on partnerships can be considerable and is likely to contribute to their ineffectiveness. This is especially evident in respect to public health challenges, none of which fits neatly within the remit of any single government department or agency (Hunter et al, 2010; Parker et al, 2010).

The report from the Institute for Government briefly considers joining up outside Whitehall by devolving power to local actors and concludes that 'the efficacy of many of these mechanisms is likely to be seriously limited so long as departmentalism at the centre remains a problem' (Parker et al, 2010, p 93). It is a conclusion supported by a report from the New Local Government Network, which studied the 13 Total Place Pilots (TPPs). TPPs were an initiative that considered how a 'whole area' approach to public services could lead to better services at less cost (Keohane and Smith, 2010). The study argued that major change was needed at the centre to break the existing top–down models and cultures of accountability and service delivery. The challenge for local areas was already considerable but was being made more difficult and undermined by current systems of funding and accountability. The clear message seems to be that more effective local coordination does not remove the need for joining up within Whitehall. Indeed, in its absence, local initiatives are likely to fail or malfunction. This was a conclusion also drawn by Gilmore (2001, p 6), who argued that 'despite the rhetoric, joint working is not happening centrally. Directives from the Department of Health to the public health community are not being heard in the Cabinet Office'. The strong message from the academic research literature is that partnerships are destined to fail if set up in a policy culture that is fragmented, misaligned and dysfunctional.

Conclusion

When analysing partnership working, a paradox is revealed: while, on the one hand, partnerships are seen to be a prerequisite for tackling 'wicked issues', on the other, they seem unable to break free from the 'silo-based' structures that govern how public services are organised and delivered. As noted earlier, in such a context, partnerships can seem like a veneer on a set of organisations and practices each with their own histories, cultures and preoccupations. It is hardly surprising, therefore, if partnerships often seem to be designed to avoid any loss of power by their members rather than effectively pooling power and resources so that the whole becomes greater than the sum of its parts.

It is perhaps not so surprising that partnerships operate in this manner since they are formed in a policy framework where government not only dictates that organisations should work in partnership, but also lays down the types of partnerships, the partnership structures and the targets they need to achieve. Thus, the room for any holistic network approaches is severely limited, as are the opportunities to try different approaches to see 'what works' or is more likely to succeed. Innovation and entrepreneurial approaches are stifled from the start.

Powell and Glendinning (2002, p 10) noted that New Labour placed:

> a 'duty of partnership' on organisations. This has been termed 'mandatory partnership working' ... or 'statutory voluntarism' in which partnership, co-operation and collaboration are emphasised and mandated at every turn.... However, earlier legislation ... shows that successful partnerships cannot be created by administrative fiat.

Administrative fiat cannot build goodwill, trust, a culture of sharing best practice and the willingness of organisations to go the extra mile for each other. Arguably, New Labour's approach to partnership working through 'mandatory partnerships' did more to stifle good partnership working than enable it. Organisations that normally might not work in partnership were forced or encouraged to work together, and were then given certain targets to achieve. In such a context, partnerships were virtually set up to fail, which may temper the appetite for any further collaborative working by organisations in the future.

As Dickinson and Glasby (2010, p 826) note in their review of effective partnerships:

> When we argue that partnership working 'doesn't work' ... this is not to suggest in any way that partnerships cannot work: more that the way they are operationalized means that they are unlikely to be successful ... because ... we have been so over-ambitious that success was never really possible.

When tackling 'wicked issues', such as those faced in public health, it is clear that this cannot be undertaken by a single agency. Just as wicked issues are complex and fluid, so hierarchical structures and a 'command-and-control' ethos will not enable local agencies to find the requisite innovative local solutions. Systems thinking and a pure network approach allow such flexibility and the room to innovate to try new approaches that are required to tackle such issues.

Whether the Coalition government can succeed where its predecessors have failed remains to be seen. Certainly, much of the rhetoric around its public health changes has centred on localism – finding local solutions to problems – and a refusal to be prescriptive from the centre, which suggests that a new approach is sought. However, it is early days and the signs are mixed that a break with the past will or can succeed. We revisit these concerns in Chapter Six after we have presented the findings from our research on public health partnerships, which demonstrate the scale of the challenge facing any government seeking to do things differently.

THREE

Public health partnerships: what's the prognosis?

This chapter reports on a systematic literature review of public health partnerships in England between 1997 and 2010 under the auspices of three Labour governments. The review was undertaken as the first stage of the National Institute for Health Research Service Delivery and Organisation (NIHR SDO) (now Health Services & Delivery Research) programme study.

As we explained in the last chapter, partnership working was a central feature of New Labour's approach to the delivery of health and social policy after 1997. A number of partnership-based initiatives centred on reducing health inequalities and improving health. Based on the literature review, which has been updated to include additional and more recent references covering the same period, this chapter considers whether these partnerships have delivered better health outcomes for local/target populations.

Public health partnerships under New Labour

Interest in partnerships intensified under New Labour and was broadened to embrace public health issues, requiring the NHS to work with other agencies in order to achieve the government's wider policy objectives (Secretary of State for Health, 1999; Wanless, 2004). Reflecting this increased interest, Glasby and Dickinson (2008) note that the word 'partnership' was recorded no less than 11,319 times in official parliamentary records in 2006, compared with just 38 times in 1989 (this is after removing references to civil partnerships, which were being debated in 2006). Indeed, more recently, Bacon and Samuel (2012) note that partnership arrangements now cover almost one third of public sector employees in Britain. As Dowling et al (2004, p 309) state: 'The message is clear.... Partnership is no longer simply an option; it is a requirement'. This is evident in the plethora of public health partnerships established during the New Labour era, including: Health Action Zones (HAZs); Healthy Living Centres (HLCs); Neighbourhood Renewal Partnerships; Health Improvement Programmes (HImPs); and Local Strategic Partnerships (LSPs).

Yet, partnerships are not cost-free. Indeed, they incur significant costs (Matka et al, 2002), and their contribution to improving health outcomes is far from clear (Dowling et al, 2004; Lowndes and Sullivan, 2004). In part, this is because the research literature on partnerships focuses predominantly on process-related issues rather than on outcomes (Dowling et al, 2004).

The Wanless Report (Wanless, 2004) on improving public health and reducing health inequalities in England, among others, noted the gap between evidence and practice in partnership working and called for evaluation to be undertaken of the emerging ways in which NHS organisations and local authorities were working together in relation to public health. Yet, this gap does not appear to have been addressed. As Glasby and Dickinson (2008, p 67) note: 'the assumption that partnerships lead to better outcomes is at best unproven and much existing partnership working remains essentially faith-based'.

This deficit in evidence is ironic given that a parallel New Labour approach to policymaking was an explicit emphasis on the need for evidence of 'what works' (Labour Party, 1997; Cabinet Office, 1999). Given the fact that in 2002 alone, it was estimated that public sector organisations were involved in approximately 5,500 different partnerships, with annual direct and indirect expenditure totalling £15–20 billion, it is curious that partnerships escaped critical assessment of their (far from negligible) transaction costs by New Labour (see Sullivan et al, 2002; Audit Commission, 2005; Healthcare Commission and Audit Commission, 2008).

Public health partnerships in England and the policy context

Under the former Conservative governments (1979–1997), little action was taken to address health inequalities. The prevailing political orthodoxy was that poverty, a major factor influencing health inequalities, was largely self-inflicted (Carlisle, 2001). However, the arrival of New Labour in 1997 palpably changed the climate. The new government attached considerable importance to public health and tackling health inequalities, appointing the first ever Minister for Public Health in England. Significant energy and resources were expended in the pursuit of innovative policy responses, notably, the partnership-centred HAZs and HLCs. Because the government had also committed itself to basing policy decisions on 'what works' many of the early public health interventions were evaluated. There exists, therefore, quite a sizeable literature on these developments, which contains lessons that remain valid.

By the second and third terms of the Labour government (2001–05 and 2005–10), it was beginning to seem as if endless successive waves of policy change and organisational restructuring were rapidly becoming New Labour's hallmark. Rather than basing policy decisions on the outcomes of research and evaluation, which the government had itself funded and commissioned, policies were being discarded 'as though they have no value once they exist' (Sennett, 2006, p 176). The government, argued Sennett, had become a consumer of policy and the latest fads and fashions and had ceased to be interested in its impact and whether it was achieving the desired results.

In addition, from 2000 onwards, the government's focus began to shift away from a broad, holistic emphasis on the social determinants of health and towards a growing preoccupation with health care issues, such as the need to reduce waiting times, improve access to beds and balance the NHS's financial books (Smith et al, 2008). Even when it did turn its mind to public health, it began to give more weight to individualistic, behaviour change interventions rather than what the government could achieve. Described as 'lifestyle drift' (Popay et al, 2010), it is a phenomenon common to many governments, even those ostensibly committed to collective action. The shift was also a reflection of the government's growing attraction to market-style thinking and neoliberal principles, which stressed individual lifestyle issues and underplayed socio-economic, structural determinants of health and the role of government in tackling these kinds of determinants (Hunter, 2007b). Such a shift was particularly noticeable in the second English public health White Paper, *Choosing health* (Secretary of State for Health, 2004; Hunter, 2005).

Throughout these various policy shifts, partnership working remained central to the government's response to public health priorities. In England, the drive to tackle health inequalities in a local context was centred on LSPs and Local Area Agreements (LAAs). Following the Local Government Act 2000, the then government actively encouraged the formation of partnership bodies and issued guidance to English local authorities in 2001 as to how LSPs should be formed. The LSPs took the form of partnerships between public, private and third sector organisations, with the aim of creating a framework within which local partners could work together more effectively to secure the economic, environmental and social well-being of their area (ODPM, 2005). The purpose of LAAs was to strike a balance between the priorities of central government and local government and their partners in reaching a consensus on how area-based funding would be used. The underlying concept behind LAAs was outcome-based and involved local government choosing up to 35 targets from a longer list of central government priorities. Local partners were then, in theory, left to decide how best to achieve these targets (DCLG, 2006; Local Government Centre, 2007).

It is against this policy context that the remainder of this chapter reports on the findings of a systematic literature review of the success (or otherwise) of public health partnerships in England.

Systematic literature review methodology

Systematic review methodology enables researchers to establish the full extent and quality of research evidence on a given question, to highlight gaps in the evidence base and thus inform the direction of future research. Indeed, in pointing to the need for better evidence on the effects of public health interventions, the Wanless Report (Wanless, 2004) on public health emphasised the importance of systematic reviews.

The systematic review synthesised empirical studies (both quantitative and qualitative) in regard to two key elements of public health partnership working: process issues (the policy levers, mechanisms and instruments in place to ensure effective delivery of public health outcomes); and outcome issues (whether these policy levers have been effective in delivering the desired outcomes).

Eighteen electronic databases were searched from January 1997 to June 2008. In addition, the bibliographies of all included studies were hand-searched and information on unpublished or in-progress research was requested via author contact. The search strategy and quality of papers reviewed are described in more detail in Smith et al (2009). The searches located 1,058 references, 895 of which were excluded at the title and abstract stage; a further 132 were excluded after reading the articles in full as they did not meet the inclusion criteria. A total of 31 references were therefore data extracted, quality appraised and included in the review. The majority of these 31 studies focused on the impact of HAZs, as they proved to be a particularly well-evaluated initiative, for which a combination of national and local studies and evaluations have been undertaken. Studies of HImPs and a range of other partnerships, including HLCs, were also identified (see Box 3.1). The results of these studies are synthesised later in a discussion that is informed by Dixon-Woods et al's (2006) critical interpretive synthesis (CIS) approach to qualitative systematic reviewing. This involves thematically exploring the theories developed in the various studies, in addition to focusing on the empirical results that are described. Most of the studies examined process, rather than outcome, issues and this is reflected in the evidence synthesis, in which there are six themes relating to process outcomes (engagement of senior management in partnerships; lack of financial and human resources; sharing information and best practice; contextual challenges; coterminosity of boundaries; and the need for 'quick wins') and only two relating to outcomes (health outcomes; and monitoring and evaluation problems). Box 3.2 highlights the inclusion and exclusion criteria used for the study and Box 3.3 explains the critical appraisal criteria for the quantitative and qualitative studies.

A further scoping study was conducted in November 2011 to January 2012 to ascertain what studies were conducted in the final two years of New Labour's period in office prior to the election of the Coalition government in 2010. Three further studies were incorporated into the review as a result of this scoping exercise in order to bring the review as up to date as possible.

Box 3.1: Main types of partnerships reviewed

HAZs (nine studies). Acknowledging the wider determinants of health, HAZs were area-based initiatives intended to develop partnership working between the NHS, local government and other sectors, with the aim of tackling ill health and persistent inequalities in the most disadvantaged communities across the UK. The first 11 HAZs were launched in April 1998, followed by a further 15 HAZs in April 1999. It was originally intended that they would last between five and seven years, but most had been wound down by 2003. The projects facilitated by HAZs varied extensively but included initiatives that aimed to address social and economic determinants of ill health, promote healthy lifestyles, empower individuals and communities, and improve health and social care services.

HImPs (four studies). HImPs are action plans developed by NHS and local government bodies working together. They were introduced in 1999 and, despite being renamed Health Improvement and Modernisation Plans in 2001, they continue to form a key approach to public health in England. The plans set out how these organisations (with, where deemed appropriate, voluntary and private sector input) intend to improve the health of local populations and reduce health inequalities. The programmes offered a three-year plan for identifying local health needs and developing relevant strategies to improve health and health care services at a local level.

HLCs (one study). HLCs were introduced in 1998 to tackle the broader determinants of health inequalities and to improve health and well-being at a local level. Funding was awarded for 352 community projects, which varied in terms of focus, ranging from service-related issues to activities addressing unemployment, poverty and social exclusion. Partnership working was an underpinning concept of HLCs. Interventions included health-focused projects (such as a physical activity outreach programme in rural localities), support programmes (such as a Community Health Information Project, which trained members of the local community to act as ambassadors for HLCs) and services (such as 'Bumps to babies', which provided midwifery and health-visiting services for young families). Although some HLCs still exist, a lack of clarity with regards to funding means that their future is unclear.

New Deal for Communities (NDC) (two studies). As part of the Neighbourhood Renewal Strategy, NDC was developed to tackle the health and social inequalities experienced by the 39 most deprived communities in the UK. In partnership with local communities, NDC seeks to address embedded issues of deprivation and long-term poverty by improving outcomes in terms of housing, education, employment and health. Interventions have mainly focused on promoting healthy lifestyles, enhancing service provision, developing the health workforce and working with young people.

National Healthy School Standard (NHSS) (one study). The NHSS was led by a partnership between the Department of Health, the Department for Education and Skills and the Health Development Agency. It had three key objectives: to raise pupil achievement; to promote social inclusion; and to contribute to reducing health inequalities.

(Also partnerships between health and local government, not a specific intervention as such.)

Box 3.2: Inclusion and exclusion criteria

Public health partnerships were defined as organisational partnerships (of two or more organisational bodies) that aim to improve public health outcomes (through population health improvement and/or a reduction in health inequalities). To be included, studies had to explicitly describe the public health partnership under evaluation or assess one of the key known public health partnerships (such as LSPs, HAZs, Neighbourhood Renewal Partnerships or HImPs). In terms of outcomes, included studies had to contain data on the impact of public health partnerships on health outcomes either directly (eg effects of partnerships, or partnership-implemented interventions, on self-reported health) or indirectly (eg by raising the policy profile of health inequalities). Studies that only involved partnerships based outside of England, and those of partnerships that were terminated by (or during) 1997, were excluded. Similarly, partnerships designed to improve clinical health outcomes, the control of infectious diseases or outcomes relating to the treatment of illnesses were not included. Opinion or theoretically based papers that did not draw on empirical data were excluded, as were studies that only examined processes of working in partnership (as opposed to public health outcomes) and non-English-language papers.

Box 3.3: Critical appraisal criteria

These criteria were used to appraise all of the included studies.

Qualitative studies
1. Is there a clear statement of the research question and aims?
2. Was the methodology appropriate for addressing the stated aims of the study?
3. Was the recruitment strategy appropriate and was an adequate sample obtained to support the claims being made?
4. Were the data collected in a way that addressed the research issue?
5. Are the methods of data analysis appropriate to the subject matter?
6. Is the description of the findings provided in enough detail and depth to allow interpretation of the meanings and context of what is being studied? (Are data presented to support interpretations, etc?)
7. Are the conclusions/theoretical developments justified by the results?
8. Have the limitations of the study and their impact on the findings been considered?
9. Is the study reflexive? (Do authors consider the relationship between research and participants adequately and are ethical issues considered?)
10. Do researchers discuss whether or how the findings can be transferred to other contexts or consider other ways in which the research may be used?

Quantitative studies
1. Is the study prospective?
2. Is there a representative sample?
3. Is there an appropriate control group?
4. Is the baseline response greater than 60%?
5. Is the follow-up greater than 80% in a cohort study or greater than 60% in a cross-sectional study?
6. Have the authors adjusted for non-response and dropout?
7. Are the authors' conclusions substantiated by the data presented?
8. Is there adjustment for confounders?

9. Was the entire intervention group exposed to the intervention? Was there any contamination between the intervention and control groups?
10. Were appropriate statistical tests used?

Sources: Rees et al (2006), Public Health Resource Unit (2006), Deeks et al (2003) and Egan et al (2007).

What does the research evidence tell us? Policy process issues

The context against, and parameters within, which partnerships operate may have a profound effect upon the impact partnerships have in addressing health outcomes. This section draws upon the predominant process issues from the literature review. As noted, many studies have tended to focus upon process issues without addressing outcomes, but, arguably, it is only through being able to contextualise partnerships in relation to the policy environment within which they operate that we are better able to understand the opportunities and barriers impacting upon health inequalities and health outcomes (Dowling et al, 2004). Otherwise, it is notoriously difficult to infer causation and conclude that partnerships have been the reason. They may have been a key factor, possibly even the decisive one, in some cases but establishing this beyond all reasonable doubt is fraught with difficulties.

Engagement of senior management in partnerships

A major barrier to successful partnership working in many of the studies was the perceived absence of key personnel with authority to act on behalf of relevant organisations within the partnership. The *Evaluation of the impact of the National Healthy School Standard* (TCRU and NFER, 2004) found that securing the engagement of senior management in local partnerships to improve the health of schoolchildren was problematic, particularly in respect of managers from Primary Care Trusts. Similarly, a study of health authorities' efforts to address inequalities in health found that: 'There was seen to be a need to gain a more general commitment to tackling health inequalities and, in particular, to ensure that senior figures were engaged in the agenda' (Benzeval and Meth, 2002, p 90). Other studies have also highlighted the need to ensure the engagement of senior management in partnerships for them to succeed (eg Arora et al, 1999; Geller, 2001). With or without the engagement of senior management, 'local champions' were regarded as crucial in some of the partnerships in order to drive the policy agenda forward (Arora et al, 1999; Speller, 1999; Benzeval and Meth, 2002).

Lack of financial and human resources

A common feature of most of the studies was that partnerships were frequently found to lack the resources (both financial and human) to adequately respond to the policy demands placed on them. A recurring issue in several studies was the lack of joint funding. Several studies reported complaints that some partners had not contributed enough (or even at all) to funding due to competing priorities on their resources (Arora et al, 1999, 2000; Bauld et al, 2001; Powell et al, 2001a; Matka et al, 2002; Sullivan et al, 2002; Benzeval, 2003; Mackenzie et al, 2003; Hills et al, 2007). In addition, commitments to contributing resources to a partnership were usually only made for a finite period of time and caused planning difficulties for several of the partnerships (Bauld et al, 2001; Matka et al, 2002; Mackenzie et al, 2003; Hills et al, 2007).

The difficulties with financial resources (particularly with the short-term nature of funding) often had knock-on effects on human resources, sometimes making it difficult to retain staff, who were wary of the finite nature of their contract, or to persuade potential new recruits to take up short-term contracts (Cole, 2003; Hills et al, 2007). Uncertainty around funding also had a number of other implications, including some programmes and activities having to be curtailed or abandoned (TCRU and NFER, 2004; Hills et al, 2007). All this created considerable uncertainty around planning for future service provision (Arora et al, 1999, 2000; Speller, 1999; Hills et al, 2007).

In respect of HAZs, the pressure to demonstrate 'success' in tackling long-term and complex health issues within a relatively short period of time meant that many struggled to set realistic objectives given the resources and time available to them, thereby placing themselves in a position where they were unlikely to be able to meet their own objectives (Bauld et al, 2001, 2005b; Jacobs et al, 2002; Matka et al, 2002; Mackenzie et al, 2003). Each of the strands of the national evaluation of HAZs concluded that a key barrier to success included the short-term (and often uncertain) nature of funding (Matka et al, 2002; Mackenzie et al, 2003; Bauld et al, 2005a).

Sharing information and best practice

Many of the studies cited the importance of sharing information between partner agencies as a key requisite of partnership working.

This involved both information concerning operational issues and the sharing of data sets (Speller, 1999; Benzeval and Meth, 2002; Freeman and Peck, 2006; Durham University, 2008). However, the studies also highlighted the difficulties and unease felt by some partners with regard to sharing information (Speller, 1999; TCRU and NFER, 2004; CRESR, 2005; Freeman and Peck, 2006). In their study of HImPs, Benzeval and Meth (2002, p 131) recount the case of one local authority encountering precisely these difficulties:

> One local authority had tried to develop a database of partner agencies' activities in order to map strategies, initiatives and good practice, and had found it very difficult to gather information from organisations. This was thought to be partly because of ... a protective approach to what they were doing, where they had achieved success and where they had failed.

A study of NDC echoed this finding, maintaining that 'silo' mentalities of partner organisations hindered the sharing of information (CRESR, 2005). Conversely, sharing best practice was seen as one of the major benefits of partnership working within some of the studies (Speller, 1999; TCRU and NFER, 2004; Freeman and Peck, 2006). One of the studies included in the HAZ national evaluation, which specifically set out to explore 'collaborative capacity', claimed that HAZs achieved at least some success on this front (Sullivan et al, 2002, 2005).

Contextual challenges

Agencies engaged in partnerships do not operate in a policy vacuum and shifting policy priorities and processes of organisational restructuring tended to have a detrimental effect on partnership working as partners had to either renegotiate relationships with new or reconfigured agencies or reorient themselves towards a new policy framework. In the case of many HAZs, both these issues had to be tackled simultaneously. Many of the HAZ studies reported that those involved in implementing HAZs believed each new Secretary of State for Health brought a new focus for national health policy and that this resulted in constantly changing priorities for the HAZs. It appears to have been partly as a consequence of these changing priorities that the future of HAZs became increasingly unclear (Benzeval, 2003; Sullivan et al, 2004; Bauld et al, 2005b). By 2000, the future funding available to HAZs was already less certain and the policy focus had shifted away from the original public health goals towards health service-related issues (Sullivan et al, 2004). By 2003, researchers found that the HAZ programme was being effectively wound down (Bauld et al, 2005a). Most of the studies of HAZs concluded that their success was constrained by this shifting policy context (Benzeval, 2003; Sullivan et al, 2004; Bauld et al, 2005a).

Similarly, in the various studies of HImPs (Arora et al, 1999, 2000; Speller, 1999; Geller, 2001; Powell et al, 2001; Benzeval and Meth, 2002), a major concern among those involved was found to lie with the restructuring of health authorities and with the consequent shift in responsibility for leading on health inequalities to Primary Care Groups (which were subsequently replaced by Primary Care Trusts). As well as causing uncertainty for the actors involved, constant restructuring required partnerships to be reconfigured and new policy networks to be formed, all of which required further effort and resources to be put into developing new relationships.

Marks et al (2010, p 67), in their study, which examined the impact of governance structures and incentive arrangements on commissioning for health improvement and on the health improvement activities of practices, note that: 'partnerships and governance arrangements were prey to constant change through reorganisations and shifts in the political agenda and this had proved a barrier'.

Taylor-Robinson et al (2012, p 6), in their study on barriers to partnership working in public health, raise the issue that:

> A key concern was that yet another re-organisation would lead to the breakup of established partnerships that have developed over a number of years. In the context of a healthy eating project, involving convenience store shops, one participant expressed concern that projects were not being re-commissioned, just at the point at which they were beginning to deliver concrete outcomes.

In addition to the unpredictable policy context, the researchers evaluating the partnerships included in this review often had to contend with the fact that a number of other area-based initiatives were rolled out during the lifetime of the partnership, with, at times, overlapping aims and objectives to the partnership being evaluated (Sullivan et al, 2002; Bonner, 2003, CRESR, 2005; Halliday and Asthana, 2005; Hills et al, 2007). Consequently, this made it extremely difficult for researchers to attribute identifiable outcomes to specific partnerships.

Coterminosity of boundaries

Many of the studies found that the requirement of some partnerships to operate with partners that had different geographical and political boundaries caused problems. For instance, the difference between local authority and local NHS boundaries posed particular problems for delivering some joint services to users. As Glendinning et al (2001, p 31) note in their study of Primary Care Groups and developing partnerships: 'differences in the boundaries of primary care groups and trusts and local authority departments continue to present problems in aligning both the planning and delivery of services'. Likewise, the case studies of three HAZs in Sheffield, East London and North Staffordshire (Benzeval, 2003) and the study of NDC (CRESR, 2005) also suggest that an absence of coterminous organisational boundaries was problematic for partnership working.

Marks et al (2010, p 67), in their study, found that in regard to the lack of coterminosity:

> This created problems in aligning priorities, providing input and manpower to local partnerships especially in areas with numerous district councils or supporting LAAs across different councils. The OSCs [Overview and Scrutiny Committees] struggled to engage all the stakeholders across such a wide area and the VCS [voluntary and community sector] described difficulties in coordinating their work across large geographical areas. Resources to cover the costs of VCS involvement were limited and the lack of an umbrella VCS body could make it difficult to coordinate views.

The need for 'quick wins'

Improving health and tackling health inequalities requires a long-term policy commitment. However, many of the HImP and HAZ studies noted policy pressure to demonstrate 'quick wins', which often worked to undermine long-term strategic planning (Arora et al, 1999, 2000; Speller, 1999; Powell et al, 2001; Benzeval and Meth, 2002; Matka et al, 2002; Mackenzie et al, 2003; Bauld et al, 2005a). As Benzeval and Meth (2002, p xi) note: 'there was a concern that performance management pushed agencies towards focusing on short-term targets, which did not sit easily with the long-term nature of a strategy to achieve reductions in health inequalities'.

What does the research evidence tell us about partnerships and outcomes?

One of the aims of the partnerships included in the systematic review was to improve public health outcomes. Yet, as noted, much of the existing literature on partnerships is primarily concerned with process issues and does not address whether partnerships are improving services or outcomes for local communities (Dowling et al, 2004). Health-related outcomes are examined here in the context of: first, whether the partnership affected health-related outcomes; and, second, if not, whether monitoring and evaluation mechanisms were put in place to be able to capture such effects in future.

Partnerships and improving health outcomes

In respect of HAZs, perhaps due to the complexities involved in these kinds of partnerships, as well as the changing policy context, six of the publications included in the review did not state whether any clear aims were being addressed and instead focus on providing descriptive accounts of aspects of HAZs or on contributing to relevant theoretical/methodological debates (Evans and Killoran, 2000; Bhatti et al, 2002; Kane, 2002; Sullivan et al, 2002; Bonner, 2003; Halliday and Asthana, 2005). Nevertheless, all of the studies do at least briefly consider the extent to which HAZs, or specific interventions that were facilitated by HAZs, might be considered 'successful' (or otherwise), and given the simultaneous emphasis on partnership working within HAZs, they therefore meet the inclusion criteria for the review. However, the way in which 'success' is constructed varies between studies, not least because the HAZs themselves appear to have varied greatly in their aims, as well as in their chosen means of achieving these aims.

In order to try to assess the possible impact of HAZs on health outcomes more clearly, two studies drew upon an analysis of data from the 'Compendium of Clinical and Health Indicators' (which is commissioned by the Department of Health and produced by the National Centre for Health Outcomes and Development). This data set 'brings together 150 indicators from several datasets including the Public Health Common Data Set indicators, population health outcome indicators, *Our Healthier Nation* indicators, clinical indicators, cancer survival indicators and others' (Bauld et al, 2005a, p 160). The HAZ national evaluation team drew on a range of indicators from this data set, with the objective of identifying whether there was a demonstrable difference between HAZ and non-HAZ areas in relation to changes in health outcomes over time. Baseline data were taken from 1997/98, the year before the first-wave HAZs, and compared with the latest available data, which was for the year 2001/02. Local authority-level data were chosen to facilitate comparisons between HAZ and non-HAZ areas. Local authorities located within HAZ areas were then compared with those in non-HAZ areas that appeared to have similar levels of disadvantage (Bauld et al, 2005a, 2005b).

This analysis produced some evidence to suggest that HAZs outperformed other areas with respect to a number of indicators related to HAZ programmes and national policy priorities (Bauld et al, 2005a). For example, positive changes in relation to all-cause mortality and coronary heart disease mortality were visible in the earlier, first-wave HAZ areas (which had had an extra year to make an impact). However, the findings were not consistent and mortality from suicide, for example, had increased in all areas, with the largest increase being in first-wave HAZ areas, even though some of these areas had prioritised suicide reduction programmes. Overall, the data employed in this strand of the national evaluation 'do not support the view that HAZs made greater improvements to population health than non-HAZ areas between 1997 and 2001' (Bauld et al, 2005b, p 436).

In contrast, three studies of particular interventions that had been facilitated by HAZs made greater claims regarding the impact of the respective interventions on local public health outcomes (Bhatti et al, 2002; Burton and Diaz de Leon, 2002; Kane, 2002). All three of these interventions involved some level of partnership working. One of these (Burton and Diaz de Leon, 2002) involved studying the impact of partnerships between the primary care services in which advice about benefits was offered by voluntary and public sector workers in primary health care settings (such as GP surgeries). The second (Bhatti et al, 2002) involved an intervention designed to provide a space in which mothers who were largely not accessing health visitor services could come together, share information and relax. The third (Kane, 2002) was a study of a project designed to engage disabled people in mainstream leisure and sports activities. All three studies reported positive health outcomes for participants but, unfortunately, the methodological approach taken by each of them was unclear, so it is difficult to assess the reliability of the findings.

In summary, the HAZ studies identified very little reliable evidence that partnership working had impacted positively on public health outcomes, although there was some evidence that it had helped broaden organisational understanding of the wider determinants of health and/

---

or push the issue of health inequalities up local policy agendas (Sullivan et al, 2002; Benzeval, 2003; Mackenzie et al, 2003).

With regard to HImP partnerships, Directors of Public Health were pessimistic as to whether their local HImP would improve public health in their districts (Geller, 2001). As Benzeval and Meth (2002, p 26) state in their study of health authorities' policies for reducing health inequalities:

> respondents who answered this question said that their HA [health authority] did have health inequalities targets. However, many of the targets cited as examples actually focused on processes or activities rather than health outcomes.... A small proportion said that they had 'tried and failed' to identify appropriate targets. Just over ten per cent said that they had no plans to develop targets in the foreseeable future.

Other studies of HImPs also found this to be the case (Arora et al, 1999, 2000). In respect of the NDC, research by Stafford et al (2008, p 301), focusing upon the health inequalities impact of the programme, found that:

> There were no consistent differences between NDC and comparator areas in the pattern of health-related outcomes for different demographic groups. In other words ... robust evidence of an NDC effect was not found, either overall or in terms of differential impacts, over and above the developments in the comparator areas.

A comprehensive longitudinal study (CRESR, 2005) also found relatively few data to support claims that NDC areas had been able to improve their relative position with regard to indicators of health outcomes.

Blackman et al (2011, pp 64, 65), in their study on local action to address health inequalities, found that too much focus on process rather than outcomes (in this context, in relation to cancer) was a concern:

> It appears that localities should avoid developing processes to excess, such as the bureaucracy of partnership meetings, writing (rather than delivering) plans and frequent monitoring. Process is not unimportant but too much focus

on plans and strategies may detract from focusing on actions that have a direct impact on the cancer gap.

Monitoring and evaluation

Part of the difficulty that many of the studies experienced in evaluating the impact of public health partnerships appears to relate to a lack of monitoring and evaluation within the partnership. For example, a study on the *Evaluation of the impact of the National Healthy School Standard* (TCRU and NFER, 2004, p 50) found that 'Although the NHSS national team were said to have spent time developing targets and indicators for evaluation, a usable set of indicators had not yet been agreed.' In the case of HAZs, even though many of the local actors involved in them were keen to produce 'hard evidence' to 'prove' the health benefits of HAZ interventions, they faced the key problem that 'relevant [comparable] data simply were not available in a usable form, as data were collected on different scales, over different time periods and with different degrees of population coverage' (Sullivan et al, 2004, p 1609).

Research by Taylor-Robinson et al (2012, p 4) found that the complexities of partnerships and the difficulties of monitoring could lead to difficulties in showing measurable outcomes:

> Underpinning the issue of complexity were concerns about the difficulty of tracking inputs and outputs over long time frames, using imperfect data, and imperfect tools. This compounded the substantial challenge of sustaining arguments for public health interventions in the face of limited resources. Some participants were concerned about the difficulties of measuring outcomes, and of ensuring that health was considered an important outcome across sectors, where partnership working may also be focussing on other outcomes, such as employment, resident satisfaction or educational performance measures.

Marks et al (2010, p 66) note of participants in their study that 'it was argued that arrangements for partnership governance lacked clarity given different systems of regulation in local authorities and it was argued that public health targets were less rigorously monitored'.

Reviewing the studies overall, the lack of indicators of improved outcomes appears to have been due to a combination of factors, including: a lack of agreed priorities; a lack of good-quality baseline data; and an absence of clear policy goals or targets (Arora et al, 1999, 2000; Speller, 1999; Geller, 2001; Powell et al, 2001; Benzeval and Meth, 2002; CRESR, 2005; Health Development Agency, 2005). It is clear that more robust monitoring and evaluation frameworks need to be implemented in future to appraise progress in partnerships. In addition, there are also difficulties in producing effective frameworks for evaluating partnerships and it is uncertain whether the impact of short-term programmes to address long-term problems, such as health inequalities, can be satisfactorily ascertained (see Dickinson, 2008).

What does the research evidence tell us about New Labour and public health partnerships?

It can be plausibly argued from the research evidence presented here that the failure of partnership-based projects to effectively achieve their aims is likely to relate to many, if not all, of the reasons set out in this chapter. Despite this rather pessimistic conclusion, New Labour's faith in partnerships remained undimmed (Department of Health, 2008b). This may seem curious given the research evidence presented here and by others (see Dowling et al, 2004). Dowling et al (2004) conclude that there is a lack of sound evidence to show that working in partnership will improve outcomes. Furthermore, a systematic review of the factors promoting, and obstacles hindering, joint working between the NHS and social services (Cameron and Lart, 2003, p 15) reached much the same conclusion, noting that:

> very few of the studies looked at either the prior question of why joint work should be seen as a 'good thing' and therefore why it should be done, or at the subsequent question of what difference joint working made.

These problems of partnerships are not confined to England. The study *Getting collaboration to work in Wales: lessons from the NHS and partners* (National Leadership and Innovation Agency for Healthcare, 2009, p 24) found that:

> Collaborative working has taken a firm root in most policy areas. However, although it continues to prosper, the evidence of its impact and success is often unconvincing. The potential benefits of this form of working – more effective use of scarce resources and better outcomes for service users – fuel the rhetoric but in practice these can

be outweighed by the costs associated with collaborative working including higher transaction costs, failure to reach consensus on purpose and priorities, and problems of converting policy intention into real action.

Indeed, in the light of the available evidence, it could be argued that partnerships established to tackle health inequalities and improve public health have clearly failed. However, the matter is not that simple. As Dowling et al (2004, p 311) note, it is important to acknowledge that:

> an emphasis on the process of partnerships may be seen as a pragmatic, albeit second best, solution ... this avoids the challenge of identifying outcomes that may take a long time to materialise and also be difficult to attribute to the partnership.

Given these problems, Glasby and Dickinson (2008, p 43) pessimistically surmise that 'we do not yet know what impact partnership working has, for whom or under what circumstances. However, the reality is that we are probably unlikely to know this with any certainty for some time (if ever)'.

Problems of establishing attribution were evidenced in several of the studies included in this review (Sullivan et al, 2002; Bonner, 2003; TCRU and NFER, 2004; Halliday and Asthana, 2005). It also appears to have been a particular concern for the national evaluation of LSPs (ODPM, 2005). In addition, partnerships have had to contend with an ever-changing policy framework, continuous organisational change, a lack of resources and, increasingly, pressure to produce evidence of 'quick wins'. It could be argued that to achieve measurable outcomes in this context is at best difficult and at worst impossible.

However, the evidence, such as it is, does offer some helpful pointers to improve policy and practice in this area. The systematic review suggests that partnerships have not always helped their cause. Problematic issues highlighted in this review, which partnership working perhaps ought to have been able to overcome, include a 'silo' mentality, that is, an unwillingness by some partners to share information or resources, and a failure to accord partnership working sufficient priority or support. Glasby and Dickinson (2008) argue that structural changes or reconfigurations of partnerships will not necessarily lead to improved outcomes. Restructuring is time-consuming, diverts human and financial resources, and can be counterproductive. This is a conclusion supported by the Healthcare Commission and Audit Commission

(2008) in their stocktake of the NHS reforms and by the Department of Health's assessments of the impact of public health policies since 1997 (Department of Health, 2008a, 2008b). The same conclusions were also reached by Wanless and colleagues in their assessment of progress in achieving the 'fully engaged scenario', namely, constant structural changes were hampering the delivery of services (Wanless et al, 2007). It was a point he had also emphasised in his public health review in 2004 (Wanless, 2004).

Despite the clear message on this score, restructuring remains in fashion and shows little sign of abating, as we shall see in Chapter Six. The systematic review also shows that robust tools to measure whether partnerships are achieving their aims and objectives through rigorous monitoring and evaluation are lacking. As mentioned, the difficulties of attribution also arise in this context and policy mechanisms to evaluate whether it is the partnership that is achieving its aims and goals or whether other policies are having an impact need to be developed.

However, most of our current thinking about partnership working falls short of what is required to make effective inroads into a series of 'wicked issues', which are often interconnected, that is, the issue of obesity, say, may be embedded in the issue of health inequalities, or the issue of teenage pregnancy may be inextricably linked to alcohol misuse. Wicked problems are invariably complex and rather messy, sitting outside single departments or silos and across systems. Yet, they are precisely the sort of problems that partnerships are set up to confront. Our review suggests that such complex, dynamic and interdependent issues have no 'correct' or 'one-size-fits-all' solutions (Edmonstone, 2010). At best, as Simon (1957) put it in his classic study of administrative behaviour, it may be a case of 'satisficing' rather than 'optimising', that is, living with the mess and making sense of it. Or, as Dowling et al (2004) note, it may amount to a 'second-best' solution. However, what this review has shown is that there are specific measures that partnerships can take to help ensure that they can succeed in working across various silos, tackling the 'wicked issues' in addressing health inequalities and securing public health outcomes.

Conclusion

Partnerships were held up by New Labour as their preferred approach to improve public service delivery across all sectors of public policy (Dickinson, 2007). Indeed, it could be said that partnerships were promoted in the New Labour era as a panacea to cure all ills. However, in the case of tackling health inequalities and improving public health, partnerships hitherto have had only a marginal impact and, on the basis of the evidence available, the cure could be said to have failed, or at least to have fallen short of expectations (National Audit Office, 2010b). As Dowling et al (2004, p 310) note: 'If "what counts is what works" ... it is uncertain whether partnerships work, and therefore, whether they should count'. However, the fact that the evidence on the effectiveness of partnerships is lacking does not necessarily mean that they are ineffective, but without such evidence, it needs to be acknowledged that the benefits attributed to this way of working are largely presumed.

Given the far from insignificant costs associated with partnerships (both in terms of financial resources and staff time) and their profusion in the New Labour era, the Coalition government (elected in May 2010), with its unexpected major reorganisation of the NHS and with public health returned to local government, offers a fresh opportunity to evaluate the effectiveness of new types of public health partnership and their ability to contribute to tackling health inequalities and improving public health outcomes. We review the changes as these affect partnership working in Chapter Six. However, before doing so, we report on the second stage of the research study we undertook into public health partnerships. Our findings provide important context and lessons for what the future holds for partnerships as the government's changes, introduced in April 2013, take effect.

FOUR

The view from the bridge: senior practitioners' views on public health partnerships

In this chapter, we consider the views of senior practitioners and their perceptions of the effectiveness and efficacy of public health partnerships. This grouping includes Directors of Public Health (DsPH), Directors of Commissioning, Councillors and other senior public health practitioners.

The research was conducted in nine locations in England between 2008 and 2010. Nine case study sites were selected according to the strength of partnership working – high, medium, low – with three sites in each category. The sample of field study sites was chosen in consultation with members of the Local Government Improvement and Development (LGID) (formerly the Improvement and Development Agency [IDeA]) Healthy Communities Team and the selection was informed by its healthy communities peer review benchmark (IDeA, 2007), in which local authorities were assessed as to how well they were tackling health improvement and health inequalities in their locality. Assessing the effectiveness of partnerships in combating health inequalities is a key element of the peer review process. As a co-investigator on the study, the IDeA/LGID's input into selecting the nine field sites was critical and we drew heavily on their deep knowledge and experience, which also had the advantage of being up-to-date in a rapidly changing policy and organisational environment.

The LGID benchmark for healthy communities is comprised of four themes: (1) leadership; (2) empowering communities; (3) making it happen; and (4) improving performance. Each of these is further divided into three key elements. The issue of partnership is an important component of themes 1 (all three elements – vision, strategy, leadership), 3 (the elements concerned with resources and delivery) and 4 (all three elements – performance management, learning culture, support) (IDeA, 2007). Our field sites in the high-partnership-based category were performing at the highest level; those in the moderate category were performing well; and those in the weak/low category were not performing as well as they might. Admittedly, these categories are somewhat subjective, being based on the judgements made by the peer review team, but the tool was validated and well-received by those subjected to it, so should be deemed a fair assessment of performance. It certainly seemed sufficiently robust to employ it in identifying the sample of field sites.

The sample of nine sites comprised local authorities and matching Primary Care Trusts (PCTs) in each category, which were ranked as follows in regard to partnership working: high-performing (sites 3, 6 and 8), moderate-performing (sites 2, 5 and 9) and low-performing (sites 1, 4 and 7). Our research findings in these sites concur with the LGID's ranking of their performance in regard to partnership working.

The phase of the research conducted among senior practitioners reported here comprised semi-structured interviews with 53 senior managers in the selected PCTs and lead elected members in the local authorities in each site. The broad aims of the study were threefold:

- to clarify factors promoting effective partnership working for health improvement and tackling health inequalities (*context-focused*);
- to assess the extent to which partnership governance and incentive arrangements are commensurate with the complexities of the partnership problem (*process-focused*); and
- to assess how far local partnerships contribute to better outcomes for individuals and populations, using tracer interventions in selected topic areas to make such an assessment (*outcomes-focused*).

These aims resulted in a number of research questions, including:

- What is understood by public health partnerships?
- Can policy goals and objectives be achieved without partnerships?
- What are the determinants of a 'successful' or 'effective' partnership?
- What barriers exist to partnership working?
- What is the impact of partnerships on health outcomes?
- What issues do partnerships face in future?

More specifically, among public health professionals, these questions became more focused and drilled down to the 'nitty gritty' day-to-day operational issues of partnership working and further issues were addressed, such as:

- What are the determinants of successful partnership working?
- What are the barriers to partnership working?
- How effective are Joint DPH posts?
- What is the impact of partnerships and joint commissioning?

- What is the role and scope of partnerships in Local Area Agreements (LAAs)?
- What is the impact of partnerships on outcomes?

The next phase of the research was conducted with front-line practitioners and service users, and the methodology for that phase is reported in Chapter Five.

What the research tells us

Successful partnership working: the key ingredients

The three factors most commonly cited by the interviewees to describe what constitutes an effective partnership were:

- a partnership that is clear about its goals and objectives;
- partners that are aware of their roles and responsibilities; and
- a partnership that has a clear strategic overview of how it is performing through robust monitoring and evaluation.

Having a clear focus about what the partnership is there to achieve was seen as essential. It was believed that unless clear goals were stated from the outset, the partnership would lack focus. Allied to this was a view that each partner agency had to be clear about their respective roles and responsibilities and that these were clear to all other agencies. This could be achieved by a partner being responsible for a specific target in the LAA, for example, or being responsible for an element of a target in partnership with others. Close monitoring and evaluation of target goals was seen as essential to ensure that progress remained 'on track', with remedial action being taken if there was a lack of progress. This respondent encapsulates some of these themes:

> "what is it that both parties are trying to get out of their relationship, so there's got to be an end, an outcome for it, and that'll govern for me whether it's successful or not, so that's key. I think once you're both clear about your desired joint outcomes, then it's about probably clarifying what you each bring to the party. You know, what is it that you can contribute and what your partner can contribute, and you need to have a good understanding of each other's statutory responsibilities and other things and strategic priorities that you're trying to achieve so you can see their perspective

whilst knowing that you're both trying to get to the same outcome. And underpinning all of that, the strategic stuff is about having good working relationships and trust, and that's people getting to know each other, as people, and spending time with each other." (Deputy Director of Commissioning, site 6)

History of working in partnership

Having a good history of joint working was seen as advantageous for a number of reasons:

- drawing on examples of best practice from the past to determine 'what works';
- although important, due to the established structures, the partnership is less reliant on key individuals as trust is built up between organisations over a period of time;
- a culture of partnership working is embedded in organisations; and
- the preceding factors bring a maturity to partnership relations.

The chair of a Local Strategic Partnership encapsulates some of these themes and the benefits a history of joint working brings:

"Oh it makes life a hell of a lot easier. I mean enormously easier. I mean I don't spend a lot of my time or virtually any of my time having to sit down and worry about some of the issues with the local PCT, such as cost shunting, and worrying about them trying to palm their problems off on us. Equally, the chair of the PCT, who happens to be an opposition councillor, you know, comes to see me regularly, she's not saying that she feels that she's got the problem of the Council trying to offload costs or problems onto them. So that immediately puts you in a good place because instead of being constantly at loggerheads over let's say cost shunting issues, which might hinder the way you go about the public health agenda, immediately we're ... happy with the way things are going so we can have a ... fairly frank and honest discussion about public health." (Site 5)

One factor that facilitated a good history of joint working was having coterminous local authority (LA) and PCT boundaries because this meant not having to work across two PCTs. A familiar factor that was found to be very disruptive to the sound functioning of partnerships was frequent structural reorganisations – often cited was the merger of PCTs and changes of key personnel in local authorities. These two respondents encapsulate some of the difficulties associated with constant organisational change:

> "I think certainly the structural changes in the PCTs where you've got people, you know, changing roles and it appears to me, certainly from the national support team visits, that where you'd got some things that were working well, they're not working as well because there's been so much reorganisation. So I think that has created quite a lot of uncertainty. It's very difficult for partners to know who to work with, and that again is probably one of the reasons where they've got fairly giant underspends because, you know, their organisations don't understand what they're doing, they haven't got a close relationship with partners." (Head of Culture, site 6)

> "I think the biggest tension has been, to be honest, within the local authority with having to go through its reorganisation, three, four, five times, however many times, because it was targeted because it was poorly performing, and quite often there that did affect partnerships. You'd bring a new chief executive in, and they would get rid of a whole tier and then bring a new one in. And then, you know, there was another fall when it became the bottom in the UK and then a whole lot of people went, a new lot in. And in some ways I'd say that forced a sort of joining of minds, but it also affected the partnership because you often, you know, you got to know people or whatever and suddenly they weren't there." (Assistant Director of Commissioning, site 4)

Loss of an organisation's 'corporate memory' meant that partnerships had to start from scratch to rebuild relationships with key personnel. This, of course, took time, and joint initiatives, in the meantime, risked losing focus as a result.

Goodwill between partners

Goodwill between partners was seen as very important in enabling effective partnerships. It engendered trust, respect, loyalty and commitment to go that 'extra mile' for each other. The following respondent explains why goodwill is so important in partnerships:

> "when I think about areas that are functioning more effectively, as opposed to areas that are functioning less effectively, I mean it's goodwill between agencies. It's also around genuine relationships between the people working, so they're working almost as if they're in the same agency, so there's a sort of shared sense of where they're going. I think partnerships that aren't going as well sometimes have a high priority but perhaps lack that goodwill or relationships to actually make that happen in a real sense, and then it just ends up on paper without genuinely moving forward." (Consultant in Public Health, site 5)

Although there was a general consensus that goodwill was essential and in some respects was seen as the metaphorical glue that holds partnerships together, there was also a recognition that robust policies and procedures, and partners being able to work together to help achieve their own outcomes, were reasons for engagement and commitment.

The role of 'local champions' and their importance

Having local champions (those individuals who strived to make the public health partnerships work) was felt to be beneficial to partnerships in a number of ways. For one thing, their commitment and passion enthuses others, which in turn attracts them into the public health arena in a variety of capacities. One DPH described how they developed programmes to identify local champions in their respective communities as they recognised the impact that they can have:

> "We've got a fantastic person now who's leading on our community engagement who really does know how to fire people up, and we've had some great events this past year to warm people up into what the issues are and to get them on board. So, yes, we had an event to launch the health checks at which 30 people signed up to be champions, and those 30 people are now being nurtured by [the individual] to help

them to know how they can be champions, what they need to do, how they can encourage other local people, etc, etc. Bring people along to health checks or take people along to activities, you know, leisure centres and all those kind of things." (DPH, site 3)

However, as already noted, over-reliance on 'local champions' can leave a partnership vulnerable if/when these people move on due to restructuring, cessation of funding, career development or other reasons.

Public health partnerships: which organisations are required?

Apart from the LA and the PCT, the voluntary and community sector, the police, various hospital trusts (eg acute, foundation, mental health), and the business sector were all regarded as crucial partners in public health. In contrast, user and carer groups and GPs were infrequently cited. Within the LA, social services, education and housing departments were the most frequently cited. When asked which agencies or sectors were not involved in their public health partnership but which they felt should be, the most commonly cited were the business sector and GPs.

Are all partners equally committed to the public health partnership?

There was a consensus that partners were generally committed to working in partnership. However, it was felt that some partners needed to show more of a commitment, and those most cited were the business sector, GPs, the probation service, the police and acute trusts. As one Director of Commissioning acknowledged in relation to elements of the NHS:

"across the PCT and the Council, I think there's strong commitment from both sides. And I think probably we are equally committed. If you were to extend this to a wider group of stakeholders, clearly I think it would be fair to say there's probably less enthusiasm amongst those parts of the NHS which are about treating ill health, because clearly they see that they really need to do their own stuff to a degree. I mean they would recognise the need for investment in public health, but they would also feel that perhaps they could utilise that money to treat people who are ill, you know, better. I'm sure there are some issues there in terms of, well, they sort of support that, but as long as it doesn't get in the way of what they need to treat people." (Site 3)

As cited earlier, it was suggested that the business sector and GPs needed more representation on public health partnerships as it was believed that they could contribute to the public health agenda in a number of ways, such as GPs acting as 'local champions' and disseminating public health messages, or through establishing private sport and fitness centres, for example, and generally being more involved in promoting public health.

Partnership working: the barriers

Various barriers to successful partnership working were identified and the key ones are considered here.

Resources and partnership working

Given that the public health function (at the time of the study) sat with the PCT, it is not surprising that many of the public health initiatives were largely funded by it. Other funding was usually drawn down from the LA or through bidding for specific initiatives. It was perceived that due to other budgetary pressures, LAs did not have significant resources to commit to public health initiatives, as a DPH illustrates:

> "They're [the LA] very strapped for cash and the PCT is in a very strong financial position, at least this year and next year, and where we've got external funding, we've had our LPSA [Local Public Service Agreement] reward grant or LAA money, what we've been doing is trying to use that to support partnership working so that if, you know, we know that the local authority won't be able to provide the funding, we've been able to use that resource to provide the funding. So there's a lot of goodwill there, there's a lot of, you know, the culture has changed." (Site 9)

In respect of pooled budgets, their existence was not extensive. Where they were referred to, it was usually in regard to mental health provision. However, partners deciding jointly where to target their resources was a more common feature, as this respondent explains:

> "I think it's true to say that we've got very few real pooled budgets. We've got quite a lot of alignment. Some of the sort

of long-standing ones, if I take mental health as an example, so improving services for mental health using the ring-fenced accounts grant that came down through the PCTs three years ago.... So although it still sort of physically sits in the two different financial systems, it's joint decisions.... So it's not pooled budgets but it's pooled responsibilities, pooled commitments for joint outcomes and so on." (Programme Director – Health Partnership, site 7)

Lack of capacity of the third sector

Although the third sector was seen as crucial in public health partnerships, and examples were given of very good health initiatives by the sector, respondents did voice concerns over its lack of capacity on a number of levels. The concerns chiefly related to smaller local voluntary organisations as opposed to large national charities, such as MIND, Turning Point and so on, and centred on the sector's ability to engage in commissioning for service delivery and on its reluctance or inability to engage strategically in partnerships. Although local authorities and PCTs, in accordance with national policy requirements, had put in place a number of measures to increase the capacity of the sector either through financial help or through providing support services, problems remained. The following respondents' comments expand on such issues:

> "it's [the third sector] not good at being able to deal with health and local authorities' means of providing services, because both local government and health are going to have to be held accountable for the funds they're spending ... and as such there has to be a lot of governance arrangements in order to make sure that money is spent appropriately. And I think a lot of the third sector find that very, very difficult ... they see themselves as a charity or do-gooders and when you start saying 'Actually you have to account for that', or 'You've got to bid for this' or something, they probably haven't got anyone in there that can put the bid together or whatever. So it frightens them off. And so that's why I think as health and local authorities we're not actually getting the engagement, and again it's something as an organisation we're looking at." (Assistant Director of Commissioning, site 4)

"I think we do work quite well with the voluntary agency both in commissioning services from them, and people like the Red Cross and Help the Aged and some of those bigger groups. What we've tried to do in the city, and it's only just happening now really, is we tried to encourage the local voluntary sector to become much more involved. And what we're trying to do as part of our procurement strategy is to make sure that there aren't so many barriers to entry for them. We've developed a market management strategy and a procurement strategy, which have been agreed by the Board, that really talk about how we can encourage local people. For sustainability and regeneration, we want to really bring local people in, but I have to say, it's not easy. We've commissioned our local CVS [Council for Voluntary Service] to work with us on developing a strategy for commissioning of the third sector in particular, and they're really keen. The bureaucracy, I'm seeing somebody this afternoon actually, the Chief Exec of the Hostel Liaison Group, to talk to her about how we would manage and work much more with the homeless community.... So they're ... keener and they have much less bureaucracy than the LA but I think the issue with them is that we don't know how to work with them very well and they don't know how to get into us, so there is something, there is a barrier between us at the moment that we're keen to break down but we're nowhere close to doing that yet. We're only at the beginning of that." (Director of Commissioning, site 1)

Are partners aware of their roles and responsibilities?

A common view was that not all partners were aware of their roles and responsibilities and, even if they were, their capacity to deliver on their commitments was questionable. LAs and PCTs were generally regarded as being aware of their roles and responsibilities, but it was perceived that some partners still saw their role in the partnership as an 'add-on' to their principal job, with little sense of ownership by some agencies. Factors cited for this lack of awareness included a lack of definition in what was expected of partners and a lack of capacity to deliver, especially by the third sector. So, although it was believed that a partner being aware of their roles and responsibilities was seen as a key determinant of successful partnership working, in practice, this was clearly not the case. As this respondent notes in regard to a lack of awareness of partners' roles and the reasons for this:

> "I think one of the reasons ... is because we've always struggled to get health onto the agenda as something that the partnerships must talk about ... because we haven't had a community strategy you see. It's basically been one of us saying 'We think health's important, would you mind discussing it at your partnership?'. And they will or they won't. One of the problems is that you've got to show somebody how they can contribute, not just in the abstract sense, but in a real sense, and I don't think we've done enough. And I think the partnership's always struggled." (DPH, site 1)

Another DPH noted the following in regard to the willingness of partners to fulfil their responsibilities: "Well I think they're aware of them, whether they actually deliver is something else. There's a subtle difference. They'll turn up to the meeting and say 'Oh yes, that's something we'll do', and then it doesn't actually happen" (site 2).

For those who believed that the partner agencies were aware of their roles and responsibilities, the main reason cited for this was that there was a good degree of ownership of targets among partners and measures such as the LAA, and a partner being responsible for a particular target clarified what their role and function was. A common theme was that the statutory priorities of an agency could sometimes distract them from full engagement in the partnership and, hence, from a partner fulfilling their role. Such priorities included an agency's own or governmental targets to be met. As one Director of Commissioning noted: "I know what I can get sacked on, and it isn't for not delivering the LAA targets. If I don't deliver on 18 weeks, I don't sign the contract at the trust, then I'm in trouble" (site 1).

However, in light of this, it was also commonly believed that more joint priorities, targets and plans were being developed through such measures as the LAA and World Class Commissioning, and it was hoped they would help more clearly to define partners' roles.

Joint Director of Public Health posts: how are effective are they?

There was a near-unanimous view that joint DPH posts were effective for a number of reasons. Predominant among these were:

- the joint DPH acted as a bridge and a facilitator between the LA and PCT;
- the post ensured that the public health priorities of the LA and PCT were joined up strategically; and
- the role helps break down cultural divisions between the PCT and LA, and with their knowledge of both the LA and PCT, this would lead to more informed decision-making.

This respondent echoes some of these themes:

> "[The joint DPH] can open doors for us. Joint policies, joint procedures, joint sharing of data, clear understanding around where there are tensions inside the council around some issues, and will that impact on us and can we ameliorate that, or do we need to put pressure back into the council in a different way, with … [the DPH] guiding us around, to make a change happen. So I think it's really beneficial to have a joint post." (Director of Commissioning, site 9)

However, there was the caveat that unless there was real commitment from both the LA and PCT to ensure that the post is truly joint, and not just in name, then its effectiveness risked being undermined.

Public health – would it be better within a local authority?

Although not a major theme, since there was no prospect of a return of public health to local government at the time of the research, respondents were asked whether the public health function should, as was the case before 1974 and is to be the case again in England from April 2013, sit with the LA as opposed to the PCT. There was evenly divided opinion on this issue in regard to those advocating the pre-1974 arrangement and those advocating the status quo. For those in favour of the public health function returning to local government, reasons given were that an LA has more influence to set the public health agenda, with schools, social services, community links and so on, and is therefore more embedded in the community. It was also believed that a PCT focused too much on a medical rather than a social model of health, whereas in the case of an LA, the social model would be predominant. For those favouring the status quo, the line of argument was that partnership working arrangements and joint posts had become more embedded in PCTs and LAs, thereby obviating the need for further change. It was also argued that such reorganisation would bring further disruption and upheaval.

Partnerships and joint commissioning

Respondents viewed joint commissioning arrangements as a work in progress. It was believed that joint commissioning was developing slowly and, as a result, at the time of the study, was not as 'joined-up' as it should be. Problems included certain partners (most commonly, councils) not being fully engaged in the process, as this respondent indicates:

> "I think they're probably about average. I came from an authority where we were much more developed in our approach to joint commissioning, joint appointments for most of the areas. [The LA has] been quite slow to develop. I think my perception is that it was reluctance on the part of the local authority rather than the PCT that's hindered progress. We have made some recent progress in terms of agreeing areas where we're developing joint commissioning more fully and so that has led to more joint appointments. We've just agreed to join our commissioners up at, well, what's tier two in the council, so a tier beneath the Director of Social Services has just agreed to join those posts. So that's quite an important step forward for us because part of the feedback we've had about why joint commissioning hasn't felt more successful or hasn't felt easier for those that have been trying to work in that way is that it's not been joined in at a senior enough level in the organisation. So we've had joint appointments working at tier four but reporting to organisations. And basically they've just been doing sort of two part-time jobs as opposed to one really well-integrated joined-up agenda." (Director of Commissioning, site 7)

A DPH also noted previous tensions between the LA and PCT:

> "Joint commissioning, I would say it's not as well developed as we would like it to be. I would say the area where it's most strongly developed would be around Children's Services, and it's been less well developed around Adult Community Care. Why? I think we didn't have the right governance structures around it. I think that there were tensions to a

certain extent between the two organisations in that the PCT was hell for leather in going for a commissioning approach to things and a sharp division between our provider function and our commissioning function. I think there was certainly more ambivalence, if you go back a year ago within the local authority, there was more ambivalence about how radical from a political point of view the council wanted to be in terms of becoming a commissioning authority rather than a big provider of services and so forth. I think there's been a lot of change in thinking about that in the course of the past year. So I would say that today the PCT and the council are much more of one mind about how we should be developing joint commissioning and we are putting in place new structures around our LSP [Local Strategic Partnership] in order to enable that. So to make it more real and less sort of lip service and to make that, in a way, the joint commissioning in particular so far as Adult Social Care was concerned was a bit of an add-on, there wasn't core business. I think we're all agreed now, and it is rapidly becoming this is the way we do business." (Site 7)

Other difficulties cited included the variability of commissioning arrangements, where they were very well developed in some areas while this was not the case in others. One respondent gives an example of this:

"on substance misuse, there are national pooled budgets. So you can't spend the money without having a joint agreement and a partnership arrangement to do that. So joint commissioning there would be much more advanced than it would be around joint commissioning for stroke services, for example. The same drivers aren't there. I think where we've got more work to do, certainly from our areas, is around older people, and that obviously is a key area for social services and for the wider local authority in terms of well-being." (Deputy Director of Commissioning, site 6)

Part of effective commissioning is having a robust Joint Strategic Needs Assessment (JSNA). Overall, it was believed by respondents that their JSNA gave an accurate picture of public health in their area, although there were some concerns over gaps in the data. A Director of Commissioning states why the JSNA worked well, but also where there were concerns over the quality of data:

"we've got our first JSNA, and it's a real picture of information and data. It was a very joined-up piece of work. The council and the PCT jointly appointed a project team to work on that, so it felt like a very joined-up bit of work. Probably, we took a view that if we only included that which we could have more confidence in, we'd have about three pages of a document. As it is, we've got 150 pages. A lot of which is very rich but is quite qualitative, quite subjective, almost anecdotal, but it tells a story and it puts that story into a single place. And I think already it is becoming the commissioning bible for commissioners in the local authority and the PCT." (Site 7)

This Director of Health and Wellbeing describes the process of compiling the JSNA and acknowledges that there are gaps:

"I think it was a really good process. I mean, I'm sure if you looked at it, there would be gaps in it. But I think it was a process where we tried to use a lot of information from the council that had already been gathered around the sustainable community strategy and those sort of things so we didn't reinvent the wheel around some of that data." (Site 3)

It was generally believed that there was adequate coordination between partners in compiling the JSNA, but there were areas of concern that revolved around the compatibility and sharing of data, as these respondents illustrate:

"the LAA targets have figured in ... terms of the commissioning strategic plan. So I think there's quite a good tie-up." (Director of Commissioning, site 1)

"I think also we've got a very strong alignment between what we've got on the LAA and what the PCT has identified through World Class Commissioning as our priorities, including within our strategic plan for the next three years and indeed for those areas which have been most challenging, the notable one I would say being teenage pregnancy and another one being the ... obesity agenda, and we have already put in additional, a fair degree of additional, resources to make sure that we, as far as possible, will deliver." (DPH, site 9)

Partnerships and Local Area Agreements

As described in Chapter Three, the drive to tackle health inequalities in a local context in England has until recently centred on LSPs and LAAs. The purpose of LAAs was to strike a balance between the priorities of central government, on the one hand, and local government and their partners, on the other, in reaching a consensus on how area-based funding will be used. The underlying concept behind LAAs was outcome-based and involved local government choosing up to 35 targets from a longer list of central government priorities. Local partners were then, in theory, left to decide how best to achieve these targets.

Have the Local Area Agreement targets been agreed by all partners?

There was near-unanimous agreement that the LAA targets had been jointly agreed by all partners. However, this did not preclude robust discussion and negotiation by partners for a particular target to be included or not, as this respondent makes clear:

> "how did we actually choose the targets that we've got? We started out with a very rigorous process, where we got the Board to agree that any targets that were coming forward for consideration for inclusion in the LAA had to be accompanied by a robust business case. That business case had to articulate a number of things, like why was this a priority ... so we had a number of tests that people actually had to satisfy. And I have to say, not all of the issues which officers from either the council, the PCT, police ... thought should be in the LAA made the final cut. And a lot of that was because they actually could not convince the Board that this was something they really wanted to do. So there was a very, it was a very strong and a very robust business case process. We had some very lengthy sessions, workshops, somebody likened it to a 'Dragon's den' where the appropriate officer had to come in and sell the case. And some of them tanked and some of them got through, but it was always evidence-based." (Deputy Chief Executive, site 9)

It was generally perceived that at the end of the process, the targets adopted by partners were agreed in a consensual manner. Disagreements centred around issues such as: which partner, or partners, were responsible for the delivery of the target; what particular target should, or should not, be included; and ensuring that the targets matched agencies' own targets, priorities and strategic plans. This respondent encapsulates some of these barriers to reaching agreement:

> "The process has been quite difficult. It's been quite difficult because initially the political stance taken by the Cabinet was that it wanted a very limited number of objectives and targets within the LAA, and it wanted to be very confident that we could deliver on them ... both within the council and among partners, the police and the PCT, particularly, were wanting many broader numbers of indicators selected within the LAA, and I was certainly arguing very strongly that I was wanting those things which were big challenges for us represented within the LAA rather than those things that we could do anyhow. So there was quite a long and quite difficult political process around what we were going to get in the LAA and what we weren't going to get in the LAA. And this was all taking place at the time of the change of the chief executive within the council as well, so it was all quite a difficult time. Anyhow, light broke out between us all. It was a good process, it wasn't a negative process, it was a process with a lot of challenges in it, but it didn't get into negativity and resentment and backbiting or anything, and we did come to a shared agreement across all the key statutory agencies with the Cabinet coming very much on board and then giving really strong leadership around making sure that we got into the LAA those issues that were a problem for the city and that we needed to do something about." (DPH, site 7)

How accountable are partners for the delivery of Local Area Agreement targets?

Respondents cited a range of mechanisms to ensure that targets were met, with lead organisations or directors or managers within a partner organisation accountable for delivering targets. However, a common theme was that processes were sometimes not robust enough to hold partners to account. This finding accords with issues reported earlier concerning the lack of awareness of roles and responsibilities, the oppressive bureaucracy in place, and the lack of an outcomes-focused approach in respect of policy delivery mechanisms. These respondents' comments describe some of the accountability mechanisms that featured in the delivery of LAAs:

> "we've got very clear delivery plans. We've got lead managers for every stream. We've got a separate performance management and monitoring stream that all partners are represented on, which we're actually strengthening at the present time to make sure the right people are there. So I would say that for partners throughout the lead agency for delivering, they are clearly aware of it and are working with those other partners who are important. So, yes, I think there's a very strong focus on delivering the LAA." (DPH, site 7)

> "each of our indicators where there was a business case that was put together [partners are] ... very clear about the ownership of it, who's the lead organisation, who's responsible for that particular theme and making sure that we're getting regular reports through the partnership, making sure that the performance is being reported through in a very timely fashion." (DPH, site 9)

As noted, there was a concern that accountability mechanisms were not robust enough to ensure that partners were accountable for delivery. This respondent's comments illustrate these concerns:

> "I was just having a discussion with one of my consultants yesterday, and one of the issues is, although they have responsibility for delivering on these targets, they are technically or officially not within the job description or necessary objectives of individuals within the council ... our ... joint public health consultant is having some issues around influencing individuals within the council to get them to play ball so that we can deliver on these agreed targets, and in a sense we were reviewing her objectives. And it almost looked like what we needed to have agreed at the outset with her was almost a work plan or an action plan specifically around influencing and engaging. Which for me, you know, I would have thought well if you've

signed off these as your targets, and you've said, you know, these are, this is how it's going to be monitored, surely some names needed to have been put in against these things so you performance manage people." (DPH, site 2)

Will Local Area Agreement targets have an impact 'on the ground'?

Two main themes emerged on this issue. First, for those who stated that targets would have an impact, the alignment of joint delivery plans and commissioning with the LAA, in conjunction with careful monitoring of targets, were seen as crucial. Second, and conversely, the lack of joined-up delivery plans, of monitoring and of ownership of targets were seen as the key factors militating against successful delivery. Overall, at the time the interviews were conducted, there was a sense of cautious optimism in regard to some or all of the LAA targets being reached, even though it would be some time before such a view could be realised. This respondent illustrates how the joint delivery of targets was an important focus of the LAAs:

> "the majority of our vital signs [targets] are in the LAA of what we've chosen. And what we did is we took the PCT strategic plan from the joint needs assessment, so we knew where our area is, and we actually targeted the 31 local authority [targets], the vital signs that are in the LAA that actually meet our strategic plan. Because that way it actually makes it easier to do joint working because you're both focused on the same thing." (Director of Commissioning, site 9)

Lack of joint delivery and a deficiency of processes and mechanisms to deliver LAA targets are highlighted by these respondents:

> "I mean, I don't feel confident or assured about any of it really, and I think that ... illustrates the point about have you got the systems and processes in place, because a part of that should be about giving you the assurance that things are working well. And I don't feel assured." (Deputy Director of Policy and Performance, site 4)

"I think that we can't work alone to try and achieve those [targets], and we need a much wider health community response to some of the issues, and at the moment, we're very separate to it. We could say we work in partnership to tackle teenage conception but, actually, city council do a bit, we do a bit, somebody else does a bit and there isn't one … team that sits there and deals with the whole lot. So I think some of them will have an impact. I genuinely believe that and I think if I didn't believe that, I wouldn't come to work. But I do think some of them are very challenging." (Director of Commissioning, site 1)

Those respondents who felt confident about the delivery of LAA targets highlighted in their delivery plans the joint nature and alignment of plans with other agencies, particularly the LA and the PCT. Good monitoring and evaluation arrangements were also highlighted as key factors to ensure the delivery of targets. On the other hand, the absence of these features was seen as the main reason for scepticism in delivering targets.

Monitoring of Local Area Agreement targets

Three themes emerged in relation to the monitoring of LAA targets:

- there were a variety of policy mechanisms for monitoring the progress of targets;
- there were difficulties at times in measuring targets; and
- more robust monitoring was required to ensure that targets were being met.

A wide variety of arrangements in regard to the monitoring of targets existed, with targets being monitored by an Executive Leadership team in one LA. Progress was then reported to the health and well-being partnership management board. In another LA, the LAA manager oversaw monitoring and evaluation; while in a third, a performance management subgroup was responsible for monitoring. Where there were named individuals or groups responsible for monitoring, it was felt that the mechanisms in place were sufficiently robust.

Another theme was the difficulty in measuring targets. This could be because of the lack of robust data or because of the somewhat nebulous nature of the target being measured, as this consultant in public health explains:

"I think looking at some of those indicators, you do find yourself thinking 'Well, I wonder how on earth they're going to measure that?' My favourite I think is the emotional and social adjustment of children in primary school, and you think 'mmm'. I forget exactly how it's worded, but you think 'Now how exactly are they measuring that?' Because that's quite a tricky one. I don't think we're using it in our mental health ... because I think we'd looked at it and thought that's a bit approximate for us. Although you could say it's relevant, but how do you measure it? You know, there are clearly people whose job it is to sit down and think about these indicators and then create them. And I have certainly been in the business of saying, in previous years, 'Okay, you've asked for this information, but actually it doesn't exist at the moment in the form that you've asked for it'. 'Oh, but we must have it.' So what you then get is varying degrees of fiction, which is of no use to anyone. And that is, what you've got there is the dislocation between people at the centre who think they know what's available and people on the ground who can tell you what's available." (Site 5)

Partnerships and outcomes

Three themes emerged on this issue:

* policy and procedures were too bureaucratic;
* the bureaucracy meant time delays were inevitable in decision-making; and
* it was believed that policy needed to be more outcomes-focused.

With a range of partners, and the amount of coordination required among them to fulfil their activities, respondents believed that a degree of bureaucracy was inevitable. With a plethora of action plans, strategy documents and meetings, it was believed that partnerships could become 'bogged down' in process issues, with the attendant danger that they would lose a focus on outcomes and become little more than 'talking shops'. These respondents echo some of these concerns:

"sometimes you sort of get a subgroup of a subgroup of a subgroup that has still got to have everybody around the table and it just becomes paralysing." (Programme Director – Health Partnership, site 7) "at the moment, everything we try and do is wrapped up in so much bureaucracy that goes back to the hierarchy and the council that it just delays everything. And that sort of encourages partnerships to break up, because I mean I'd be the first to say 'Oh don't bother, just let's do it, let's just get on with it, otherwise we're never going to get anywhere, because it will take us six months to go that route, if we do it ourselves we can do it in three'. So that's the biggest sort of knock on partnerships that there is really, when you know things are going to be delayed so much." (Director of Commissioning, site 1)

Given the complexity of the policy process and the difficulties in ensuring that partner agencies were aware of their roles and responsibilities, it is perhaps unsurprising that respondents believed that, as highlighted earlier, a large amount of goodwill between partner agencies was the 'glue' that held partnerships in place and enabled them to overcome the barriers they faced.

Could health outcomes be achieved without partnership working?

The near-universal response on this issue was that health outcomes could not be achieved in the absence of partnerships. There was recognition that because public health issues are multifaceted and complex, a strategic and joined-up approach was needed to tackle these commonly termed 'wicked issues'. There was also the view that individual agencies did not have the capacity to deliver public health improvements on their own and that it was only through combining resources and having a joint delivery strategy in place that agencies could together make an impact. These respondents illustrate some of these points:

"we don't have the capacity, and I think there's something about what other partners bring. Because we always wear the health hat, but the local authority brings education, employment, loads of other things and the voluntary sector bring a whole different perspective too, and a partnership is about joint working, it's not one person doing it all. It's a bit like a marriage really. So there is no one solution to these problems, to these health inequality public health problems." (Director of Commissioning, site 9)

"If you mean without partnership by working in separate silos we can achieve those goals, I think that's exceedingly unlikely." (Consultant in Public Health, site 5)

Are outcomes delivered by the partnership?

Respondents were questioned as to how they could be sure that it was the partnership that was having an impact on the delivery of targets and agreed outcomes as opposed to an individual agency. Three themes were predominant:

- respondents did not know if it was the partnership that was responsible for the delivery of outcomes as this would be difficult to measure or quantify;
- through the accountability mechanisms in place, it could be seen which agencies were delivering; and
- as long as the desired outcomes were achieved, it did not matter whether they were delivered by the partnership or not.

On the issue of respondents not knowing if it was the partnership that was responsible for the delivery of outcomes as opposed to a single agency, since this would be difficult to measure or quantify, the following respondents consider the difficulties:

"how do you know whether it was the partnership that delivered it? And the only way you could really test that is to ... apply the definition of causality to the outcome, which would be slightly difficult, wouldn't it, because you could ... go for a major impact on, say, all age all cause mortality and have a chance occurrence of a real drop in the number of deaths for some reason, and you would never know that." (Deputy DPH, site 8)

"we need to first be clear about what's bringing about the changes in our outcomes. I'm not sure we're clear enough. Take teenage pregnancies, you know, there's about four or five key strands to that programme, and we see an improvement, but I'm not sure we could say which one of those four or five strands was delivering that improvement. Some of it relies on the partnership, some of those don't, but it would be quite hard to isolate whether it was the partnership that was giving them success." (Director of Commissioning, site 7)

There was a belief that the partnership was responsible for the delivery of outcomes and this could be identified through robust monitoring and accountability mechanisms. Although less predominant, there was also a view that the partnership acted as an enabler for the delivery of outcomes, as these respondents make clear:

> "I suppose it's by being clear from the outset what contribution each has to make. I think sometimes people just think by getting around a table they can achieve something rather than working through those assumptions. So being clear about what it is that you're trying to achieve, ultimately, the outcomes you're aiming for, and if that's the outcome, what are the preconditions that you need to achieve it. When you start really breaking down what the preconditions are, sometimes it becomes clear which are the agencies and partners that will have the biggest impact on that precondition. So I think if you've done that work beforehand, it is easier to measure whether the partner is playing the role they're supposed to make. But quite often people don't do the pre-work." (Deputy Director of Commissioning, site 6)

> "My view is as long as you're delivering the outcomes, I would always argue that an enabler to that would be the partnership because the partnership outcomes are that you've got a much wider – you've got the resources of both organisations that can help you to achieve things and you've got a much better strategic tie-up so you haven't got two organisations fighting against each other." (Director, Health and Wellbeing, site 3)

There was a view that it did not matter if the partnership did not deliver the outcome as long as the outcome was delivered:

> "As long as you're agreeing between you what the metrics are, what the baseline is and what you're measuring, and you agree between you that that's what's going to, if you see a shift, that's going to be success, then I think that's

probably as good as it gets, isn't it?" (Director of Civic Engagement, site 8)

"I'm not actually that fussed about whether it's the partnership that delivers it. I think, you know, it's a bit apple pie." (Director of Commissioning, site 5)

Given the differences in opinion over whether partnerships could be identified as the essential ingredient for achieving tangible health outcomes, it may come as no surprise that it was argued that better monitoring was required in terms of partnership delivery to see 'what works'.

Cost–benefit analysis: are the resource costs of partnerships justified in terms of outcomes gained?

As highlighted in our literature review, given that partnerships are not cost-free, since they incur significant resource costs (both capital and human) to establish and maintain, respondents were asked whether they felt that partnerships justify these costs in terms of the outcomes gained. A qualified 'yes' was the most common response to emerge, with respondents believing that partnerships do justify their transaction costs in terms of outcomes gained. However, as indicated, this view was qualified by a number of caveats.

First and foremost among the reasons in support of partnerships, respondents believed that with agencies working together, partnerships removed duplication and channelled resources more effectively. There was also a view that partners such as LAs and PCTs would be working on common themes to improve public health and it therefore made sense for them to do it together for the aforementioned reasons. Partnerships were also seen as more successful in leveraging resources for specific initiatives rather than leaving it to agencies acting alone. There was also the recognition that some public health issues were complex and multifaceted, requiring a coordinated approach by different disciplines since they could not be tackled by an individual agency. Therefore, agencies had to act in concert to address these issues. These respondents are representative of these views:

"I think what we do know is in learning to work together across boundaries, we are aware of lots of duplication that's gone on over the years which can only represent major wastage of resources, and things that we've done for years that haven't had an impact either. So you could argue that the learning that comes from, you know, learning to work in partnership because we know more about who's doing what and why and how, we should have the capacity to provide more value for money at the end of the day and better impact. Whether we do or not remains to be seen, but we should because we do know more now and we do know that we are doing some crazy things and have been doing crazy things for years." (Strategic Director Children and Young People Services, site 7)

"For something like smoking, it's easy because it's such a huge issue and by far the most important health inequalities issue in the city – you know, 500 people a year die of it, 50% of our health inequality is smoking. There can be no doubt that [it] is the ... most important thing of all, and because of the scale of the task, it has to be a partnership agenda. It cannot be done, almost irrespective of the cost–benefit ... however much time I'd have to put into that, I would put it in because, in the end, it's the most important thing I can deliver. Now that's knowing that the intervention or knowing that the effect of the outcome has such a beneficial effect on health." (DPH, site 1)

In relation to smoking cessation, a DPH argued that the health benefits for the population far outweighed the costs of partnership and asked the rhetorical question: 'what is the cost of getting a smoking quitter?' (site 8). In other words, the possible savings from a person stopping smoking and the health benefits to that individual and the potential savings on treatment by the NHS outweighed the costs of partnership. There was also the argument cited that the multifaceted issues involved in tackling health inequalities meant that only a partnership approach would work.

As mentioned, although respondents by and large believed that the value of partnerships did outweigh their transaction costs, there were a number of caveats. Predominant among these was that the partnership had to be seen to be delivering on its agreed outcomes otherwise its costs were not justified. These respondents echo these concerns:

"I don't think partnership working is de facto a good thing. It is only a good thing if it delivers results, outcomes, whatever you want to say. And in some senses the test of the new Health and Wellbeing Board will be delivery of the LAA targets and other things." (Strategic Director of Health and Adult Community Care, site 7)

"Well, I suppose … it all comes back to what the aim of the partnership is, if the vision's there and does it deliver it? If it doesn't deliver what you want, and it just becomes a talking shop, and I've been on many groups like that, where it just, they're not cost-effective and they're not a good use of anyone's time or anything. Where there is a clear vision and a clear outcome, they can often be very cost-effective." (Assistant Director of Commissioning, site 4)

What public health outcomes have been achieved through partnership working?

Respondents were asked what particular initiatives had been successful in tackling health inequalities and improving public health through working in partnership. Two main themes to emerge from the interviews were: first, that the partnership was on track to deliver on a variety of public health outcomes, but that these had not as yet been achieved or may not be achieved; and, second, that discernible outcomes had been achieved through working in a collaborative manner.

A variety of projects in the public health arena were cited to demonstrate the value of partnership working, with alcohol reduction, smoking cessation, obesity and teenage pregnancy to the fore. These respondents give a representation of where they believe outcomes (against projected targets or delivery plans) had not been achieved hitherto but were on course to be:

"Okay, go with teenage pregnancies. If we hadn't worked with the local authority to help get the school nurses into the schools and to start dealing with sex education and giving out contraception and being available, we would not be on the road to sorting out our teenage conception targets. We couldn't have done it alone because this had been going on for years … and I'm told the headmasters were very reluctant to have nurses in the school who did anything but nursing. You didn't do health education or public health stuff at all. It's only by starting to do the local partnerships that this is being addressed, and we're starting to see a difference for those girls." (Director of Commissioning, site 9)

"teenage pregnancies is one where the will is there, the partnership is there, but the facts on the ground tell you that the message ain't getting through, and we've got to try and think of where we can sort of move on and work better." (Chair of LSP, site 9)

This respondent identifies where they believe discernible outcomes had been achieved through working in partnership:

"I think there is good evidence that the partnerships do deliver. So, for example, teenage pregnancy is a good one, where we've got a ... teenage pregnancy partnership, which is hosted through the ... [LA] with good health buy-in, and the one area that they really focused on and did a lot of work on the ground, so almost community development-type role of going out and finding out what people wanted and needed and then commission that, we can show that that's really had a major impact on the rate in that local district. And what we're doing now is making sure that we're replicating that same sort of process in the other districts to emulate the reduction in teenage pregnancy.... I guess another one ... would be healthy schools, which is a county target but we've put in the staff on the ground to support the delivery of healthy schools in each of our schools. With good success, I mean we're pretty much ahead of the national targets now on delivering healthy schools." (Deputy DPH, site 8)

Discussion

As we have noted, little is currently known about public health partnerships despite the fact that collaborative working is a key competency of public health practice and partnerships remain firmly on the Coalition government's policy agenda. Even less is known about how effective partnerships are in achieving public health outcomes and tackling health inequalities.

From the first round of interviews reported in this chapter, although partnership working was regarded as the only or preferred way to tackle the multifaceted nature of health inequalities and deliver improved public health outcomes, there was a clear recognition that working in partnership was not unproblematic. Partnerships were often seen as too bureaucratic, with not all partners aware of their roles and responsibilities. This was sometimes combined with poor policy and management mechanisms to hold partners to account. Even though LAAs were designed in part to ensure an approach focused on outcomes, it is clear that this has not universally been implemented, with evidence of a lack of delivery mechanisms to ensure that policy is outcomes-focused. Policy and procedures need to be more streamlined, with an emphasis on outcomes rather than on the policy process itself. As has been shown, those partnerships deemed to be successful were those in which the policy processes were outcomes-focused, with joint delivery mechanisms, clear lines of accountability, the full engagement of relevant partners and careful monitoring. Conversely, less successful partnerships were deemed to be deficient in respect of these key features.

It is important, therefore, that agencies are aware of their role and function within the partnership and that their responsibilities in achieving agreed objectives or targets are clearly set out. It is also essential that the objectives or targets adopted by a partner closely align with their own targets, priorities and delivery plans, as this avoids duplication, streamlines delivery and ensures a 'win–win' scenario for both the agency and the partnership as a whole.

Although, the former government's emphasis was on targets, as has been seen, there is a danger that targets can both encourage a short-term approach to the policy process and reinforce a silo mentality among agencies, thus rendering partnerships less effective than they might otherwise be. Targets can also tempt partnerships (consciously or otherwise) to focus on 'quick wins' and target the 'low-hanging fruit' in regard to policy priorities.

Joint posts have been claimed to be a valuable aid to partnerships, which help bridge the gap in terms of policy delivery and facilitate joint working between LAs, PCTs and other partners. We comment further on these posts in subsequent chapters.

The absence of pooled budgets has arguably militated against delivering policy outcomes and more pooling of resources, together with partners identifying joint targeting of resources for specific initiatives, would perhaps contribute to the improved delivery of outcomes. However, a report by the Audit Commission in regard to joint financing across health and social care found little evidence that pooled or aligned budgets had much impact on influencing outcomes across a variety of health and social care settings (Audit Commission, 2009).

Joint commissioning is still seen as 'work in progress'. More of it is perceived to be needed to improve public health outcomes, particularly with relevant council directorates and other key stakeholders, including the voluntary and community sector (although issues of capacity in this sector need to be recognised). It is also apparent from many of the interviewees, including DsPH and Directors of Commissioning, that commissioning has to be more closely aligned to key delivery plans, such as local authority corporate plans and community strategies. To aid commissioning, JSNAs need to be able to give a more comprehensive picture of local health needs and a key part of this is through ensuring that the various agencies' data are more compatible to enable sharing. It is clear that much good work has been done and needs to continue in engaging smaller local voluntary and community sector organisations in public health partnerships where they are perceived to add value.

Our research shows that through bodies such as LSPs, and initiatives such as the LAA, together with their alignment with corporate plans and community strategies, there is a danger of partnerships (already complex by their very nature) becoming too weighed down through burdensome and cumbersome processes and structures to be effective. Chapter Five considers partnerships from the other end of the spectrum and discusses the way that they are constituted and delivered by those practitioners working on the front line of public health. It offers conclusions in regard to the contrasts in the methodologies and approaches to partnership working from those at strategic and front-line levels, respectively, and lessons for public health partnerships overall.

FIVE

The view from the front line: practitioners' views on public health partnerships

This chapter focuses upon the research findings of the second phase of the study with front-line practitioners and service users. The interviews were based on the selection of four 'tracer issues' in four of the nine locations reported on in the previous chapter. Topics were chosen that were of high priority in those areas' Local Area Agreements (LAAs), namely: obesity (site 2); alcohol misuse (site 1); teenage pregnancy (site 4); and smoking cessation (site 3). These public health issues have been identified in order to explore through interviews with front-line staff and focus groups of service users their perceptions of partnership working. Although the context for partnership working will be different in future, it is unlikely that the views expressed have lost their salience since, for the most part, they transcend particular structural configurations.

Methods

A total of 32 semi-structured interviews were conducted with practitioners in the four study areas, and four focus groups in three of the study areas were held in regard to three of the tracer issues: obesity, alcohol misuse and teenage pregnancy. For the most part, practitioners were front-line staff responsible for delivering service provision in the selected tracer issue areas, but there were also some middle managers included in the sample.

The aim of this phase of the study was to address a number of key questions in relation to public health partnerships, including:

- What are the perceived benefits of partnership working?
- What are the determinants of successful partnership working?
- What are the perceived benefits of partnerships for service users?
- What are the views of service users towards partnership working?

Benefits of partnership working

Our interviewees were unanimous in their view that there were many benefits to be gained from working in partnership. Chief among these was having a coordinated approach to the delivery of services, the benefits that networking with partner agencies can bring and agencies bringing different perspectives to working in partnership on complex, multifaceted issues. In addition, having shared agendas and resources and promoting shared expertise were also believed to be key benefits of working in partnership, which are evidenced throughout this phase of the study.

A coordinated approach

A major theme of the benefits of working in partnership was being able to act in a coordinated manner with other agencies. It was believed that acting in such a manner brought the benefit of each agency's perspective to bear on tackling a facet of a public health issue in accordance with their particular knowledge and expertise. It could range from one agency tackling the prevention agenda in teenage pregnancy to another agency offering advice and support to would-be teenage mothers. Having a coordinated approach was also claimed to be cost-efficient and effective. This could be through pooling resources or coordinating publicity campaigns to ensure the effective and efficient targeting of messages to the intended audience. It was also believed that given the complex and multifaceted nature of public health issues ('wicked issues' as we have referred to them), no single agency could tackle these problems alone and that a coordinated approach was therefore required. The following respondent exemplifies these points:

> "I could be spending a lot of money on making sure that GPs are identifying alcohol misuse and referring appropriately, but then if ... we're granting licences to every single place that wants to open up a new bar and, you know, just allowing people to get increasingly drunk in the city centre, it's almost defying the point of it really. So I think working together can give a better overall approach to alcohol, because we've all got the same sort of aim, so I think that's really positive." (Public Health Consultant, site 1)

However, the main benefit of a coordinated approach was seen to lie in offering a more tailored and seamless service for service users themselves. With such an approach between agencies in place, service users would have more integrated packages of care and provision and where one agency could not offer one aspect of provision, users could be referred to a more appropriate agency (the experiences of users is discussed later). These pathways of care and provision were regarded as one of the major benefits of working in partnership. It was also believed that those in hard-to-reach groups would benefit by perhaps accessing one service and then being encouraged and signposted to use other services. The signposting argument is illustrated by a smoking cessation advisor:

> "So, in fact, what I'm offering is a stop smoking service, but what I'm also offering is 'Why don't you join this health training programme? Why don't you go on this walk and … get the health check?'. So even though that takes me a few seconds, I'm throwing them in, and a lot of the time they'll go 'Yeah, you know what, I am interested in that, shall we fax off a referral'. And it's all the little things like that, having the knowledge like that, and they do it for us as well, so it works both ways, and it's giving a better health outcome for the residents." (Site 3)

It was believed that a coordinated approach also gave the service user more choice in the services they could access in terms of what was most appropriate in meeting their needs. Also, given that a user may have a number of health and other related issues to deal with, the multi-agency approach was essential in addressing these. One respondent gives an example:

> "The benefit for them is that they do get a more … [seamless] service; they're not passed from pillar to post. They have an identified worker that can sort of vouch or say 'I work with this health visitor, she's really good', and it's a bit of reassurance for the young person, so they're more likely to engage with another service because they've got a contact point or a worker or a bit of encouragement to go. And I think they're more likely to engage and get a better service and get more access for the things that are out there. So they'll be less isolated and their children would be less isolated and more willing to progress on to different things, such as maybe education … as a result of that. And I think it opens a lot of doors for them as well if they can

see what help's out there, whether it's a health issue or a
housing issue or a confidence issue because … if they have
a positive experience with one agency they're more likely
to go on and work with another." (Young Parents Personal
Adviser, site 4)

Networking

Study respondents believed that one of the key benefits and successful
determinants of partnership working was networking. Networking
could range from informal or formal partnerships with agencies to
arranging training and joint meetings to discuss policy and strategy.
It was believed that networking could, by its very nature, lead to
further beneficial partnerships being forged. Networking also allowed
agencies to see where their respective agendas and priorities aligned
and how they could assist each other and, more importantly, service
users. Through networking, service users could be referred to the most
appropriate agency. Furthermore, networking enabled the profile of
agencies to be raised, not only among professionals, but also among
service users. A further benefit was that through regular contact,
professionals were kept up to date with the latest policy developments
locally and nationally. A Health Improvement Coordinator illustrates
some of the benefits of networking:

> "half [of] my role is putting people together, people who
> need to meet each other, so it may even be my role would
> just be introducing one partner to another partner in a
> particular project. So network[ing] is really important
> because you get to have a bit of continuity with what you're
> trying to [do], and there's a lot of the left hand not knowing
> what the right hand is doing, and so it becomes streamlined,
> it makes it more efficient and more effective, more value of
> money, better value for money." (Site 2)

Different agency perspectives

Having different agency perspectives coexisting in a partnership
was viewed as beneficial. Allowing agencies to give their particular
viewpoint on a policy problem or issue was important because the
issue or problem was then viewed from multiple angles and a more
rounded, holistic approach enabled a more satisfactory resolution of
issues and the search for innovative solutions. Furthermore, other

perspectives challenged the preconceived views of each agency, which was seen as helpful. The perspectives of other agencies could also change the behaviour of how an agency operated in relation to policy formulation or implementation. This could be, for example, a slight change in operational procedure prompted by the suggestion of a partner. A Specialist Midwife in Teenage Pregnancy echoes the views of many respondents:

> "So I do think that other agencies pick up on different elements ... because they're working with them [service users] perhaps in a different way to how maybe I am, you know, they see certain different things that ... obviously are very important really and can have a very dramatic effect on the outcomes ... for that young person." (Site 4)

Shared expertise and resources

A claimed benefit of partnership working was the ability to draw on each agency's expertise and skills. It was believed that this brought major benefits not only to the agencies themselves, by expanding their own understanding and skills, but also to service users, with the existence of a range of professionals to draw upon for support. These two respondents illustrate these views:

> "we have a programme of sex education that we deliver in Year 9 in our secondary schools ... which is a multi-agency team, so it has strengths of different professionals. So those young people are benefiting from a very broad range of professionals really. The skills of youth workers who can communicate better than perhaps health professionals can. But equally we've got health professionals working in partnership as well so that if any of the questions that come up from the sessions are health-related, we've got the appropriate people then that can answer those questions. But, equally, we've got the skills of youth workers who are able to tease out issues that young people may want to discuss." (Teenage Pregnancy Coordinator, site 4)

> "you can't do it on your own; no one agency could do it on their own. I mean everybody specialises in their own skills and if you think that you're the one agency that's got all the skills, you'll fail because you haven't, you know, none

of us have. With working in partnership, the families just get every bit of information and service support, because everybody specialises in their own areas." (Children's Centre Coordinator, site 4)

Sharing resources was regarded as beneficial by respondents and could range from the free use of a hall for an event and producing information leaflets jointly, to shared training events.

What makes a partnership work?

A number of issues can determine whether a partnership is successful or not. Some of these may be under the partnership's control (ie how well they share information) and some may not (ie organisational change imposed from above and resulting in the breaking up of networks). This section focuses upon what were deemed by respondents as the key factors that could aid or impede successful partnership working.

Sharing information

A major theme was that despite the predominant view that there was good sharing of information by partners, a significant minority believed that information sharing was either a mixed picture at best, or poor at worst. For those who cited good information sharing between agencies, this assessment was usually predicated on protocols for sharing information being in place and agencies keeping each other up to date in regard to policy and practice issues. Regular meetings, networking and shared training arrangements also facilitated the sharing of information, in addition to the use of dedicated email groups. This respondent echoed some of these themes in relation to having information-sharing protocols in place and good information sharing between agencies:

> "Every one of our clients when we first work with them has filled in a shared information consent form, which then is produced if requested by another service. For an instance and scenario, perhaps one of the agencies that, let's say Jobcentre Plus, we are required at times to obviously, you know, send a fax over and show them the shared information consent because, you know, we're ringing up about young people's benefits, it could be anything." (Young Persons Personal Advisor, site 4)

For those who believed that information sharing was mixed or poor, there were a number of reasons for this: lack of information-sharing protocols in place; confusion over what information can or cannot be shared, particularly around service users; and issues of data protection. In addition, and more generally, poor communication between agencies was cited as a reason. Two respondents illustrate many of these themes:

> "I think what happens is that a lot of clinicians on the ground get very confused between issues of confidentiality and information sharing, and I think that that can be a real barrier sometimes. I think that we are pushed and pulled in so many directions. We're often criticised, for example, when there are inquiries, like serious case reviews or anything, for not necessarily being proactive in sharing information. And I think sometimes that two-way street simply doesn't happen because people, workers on the ground, are not clear about what their issues around confidentiality and consent and data protection are. I think it's a very, very complex subject really I think." (Dual Diagnosis Clinical Director, site 1)

> "I think probably that we're not always clear sort of what's going on with the City Council and ... Probation and Social Services and so on, and who to share what information with." (Clinical Lead, site 1)

How important is goodwill in the successful functioning of partnerships?

A near-universal consensus was that goodwill, as mentioned in Chapter Four, was 'the glue' that kept partnerships together and functioning effectively. The importance of personal rapport and friendship between partners was echoed time and again in interviews. Respondents cited goodwill, trust and a shared passion in achieving better public health outcomes as the principal features in cementing and driving partnerships forward. A Specialist Public Health Nurse explains what goodwill means in practice:

> "I'd say that relationships are key because if you get somebody that you have difficulty having a relationship with in a partnership agency, then it's ... going to be very difficult. And I think forging relationships with the other agencies was key, and the staff on the ground, the actual

smoking advisers, their relationships with other agencies is
key.... Because we have got good relationships with other
agencies here ... and I do know that if I phoned up today
on behalf of the smoking service, if I phoned up, say, the
substance misuse or sexual health and said 'Look, you know,
there's this young person coming down tonight' or whatever,
you know, they would wait for them, they would go the
extra mile for them, as would the smoking service." (Site 3)

Another respondent outlined why personalities can be key in
partnerships:

"I think government fails to recognise that partnerships
are made up of people, and not positions. Not sort of
appointments, they're made up of people. If people don't
get on, partnerships will fail. And people get on when they
get benefit out of something." (Joint Consultant in Public
Health, site 2)

In addition to goodwill, the role of local champions to drive agendas
and partnerships forward was also seen as very important in the multi-
agency framework.

'Local champions': driving the partnership forward

Local champions – those individuals with the drive, passion and
commitment to move the agenda on – were regarded as very important
in partnership working. On the front line, they were the people who
developed networks, spread good practice and helped coordinate policy
and practice in a partnership. Having good policy and procedures was
not deemed to be sufficient or even adequate without there also being
the people on hand with the drive and commitment to make policy
commitments a reality within the partnership. A respondent explains
the importance of a local champion in the context of what happens
when they leave:

"certainly we've struggled for a long time now having to
champion teenage pregnancy to be fair, and we ... were
successful in finding somebody. He was really taking it,
you know, we were making real good progress ... because
he was really sort of pushing all that work sort of forward.
So we've had to sort of revisit that, again, and it lost its

momentum for a while I think, as like new things do when new people take over who perhaps don't always have that as their main interest if you like." (Specialist Midwife in Teenage Pregnancy, site 4)

Organisational change and the effect on partnerships

Views were split on the effect of organisational change on partnerships. First, there were those who had no opinion or did not think that it was an issue, either because they were not affected by a particular reorganisation, for example, or because they worked in the community or voluntary sector or at a level where it would not impact on their role in the partnership. Second, there were those who had been affected by organisational change, either within their own or partner organisations, who believed that it did have an adverse impact on partnership working. The main reasons they cited were the loss of key personnel, the breaking up of partnership networks and the loss of an organisation's 'corporate memory' as a result of a merger or reorganisation. The following two respondents elaborate on these themes:

> "the memory of an organisation is invested in the people that work in it. If you constantly change the organisation and the people, the organisation ... will never have a memory, no matter how well you file the paper, because people ... think differently, so they won't file things in the same places." (Joint Consultant in Public Health, site 2)

> "Recently, there have been some mergers of things and it stops things for a while because everybody is trying to figure out where they stand, where they are ... and ... you have to build up new links and new contacts, so any mergers and moves does cause a disruption, it's bound to, and they do." (Area Manager, Probation Service, site 1)

Could public health be delivered without working in partnership?

We asked if public health aims and objectives could be achieved in the absence of partnership working. Not unexpectedly, a resounding 'no' was the near-unanimous response. Most respondents felt that because of the complexity of issues such as alcohol reduction, teenage pregnancy, tackling obesity and smoking cessation, they simply could not be tackled by one agency acting alone. As noted earlier, it was believed that a coordinated approach based on the utilisation of different resources and skill sets was required to tackle these issues. In addition, the sharing of resources and expertise also meant that more help and support could be provided to local populations than would be possible in respect of organisations working by themselves in silos and, most likely in the process, duplicating effort.

Although we have so far documented the benefits and the determinants of successful partnership working, this is not to suggest that partnership working does not have its barriers or problems, which come at a cost. It is to these that we now turn.

Barriers to partnership working

Major themes that emerged in relation to barriers to partnership working were the different priorities of the various agencies, partners not being aware of their respective roles and responsibilities, and duplication of provision.

Different priorities of agencies

An agency's statutory priorities, an agency not seeming to share targets and priorities with other organisations tackling a particular public health problem, or an agency being inward-looking and only engaging with its own priorities were seen as the principal reasons for organisations not fully engaging in partnerships. One respondent exemplifies some of the difficulties encountered in engaging with other agencies:

> "the other services actually considered that smoking was kind of low on the priority. That a bigger priority would be sexual health or substance misuse and then smoking came last, and part of my role was saying to services actually 'No', you know, 'Smoking kills!', do you know what I mean, and quoting the document Smoking Kills and other documents and saying actually, you know, it is just as important and if somebody is smoking cannabis and using tobacco, yeah they need substance misuse but they also need follow-ups in the smoking cessation service as well because they're smoking tobacco. And if they work jointly, then that works, that's fine. But I think, yeah, I do think that maybe other services didn't understand it, but also it wasn't a priority for other services. And also, for other services, like say a GP practice,

young people aren't necessarily the priority." (Specialist Public Health Nurse, site 3)

Partnerships: roles and responsibilities

It could be said that there was a general response of 'maybe' in regard to whether partners were aware of their respective roles and responsibilities within partnerships. Although some respondents believed that partners were fully aware of their roles and responsibilities, a more common finding was that they were either unaware, or only partially aware, of them. A number of reasons were offered for this and no particular themes predominated. Three respondents give instances across the spectrum of partners' awareness of their roles and responsibilities:

> "we do a lot with children services, then of course as you know where there are care plans, then it's quite specific and written and black and white as to whose role and what piece of work that agency's doing; perhaps not so much with the ones that aren't working with children services. But I think because of service level agreements within all those agencies, say we have one with Jobcentre Plus, they're well aware of their roles and responsibilities, and we're aware of ours." (Teen Parents Personal Advisor, site 1)

> "It's a work in progress. We are getting there, yeah. We've been doing a lot of work on alcohol in the last little while and, yeah, we are getting there but we're not quite there yet, no." (Clinical Lead, site 1)

> "I think the most practical [barrier is] just trying to find the time to ... create the meetings, time to move forward the actions from meeting to meeting, sometimes ... it can be a little bit ... some groups end up doing more of the work than others, so there's not such a fair distribution. Sometimes, there's a challenge that it's kind of whose responsibility is it to kind of carry forward the project as a whole." (Public Health Nutritionist, site 2)

Duplication of services

One of the claims made for partnerships is that they can help avoid duplication and are a useful tool for mapping provision in an area.

Respondents were asked how far duplication of services was an issue in their locality and whether it was a good or a bad thing. The consensus view was that there was no, or very little, duplication of services and what there was need not be regarded as a bad thing. A Joint Consultant in Public Health highlights how partnerships help to avoid duplication:

> "I think partnership work is really helpful in avoiding duplication. We've just had a discussion ... about this lifestyle proposal, and part of it is a telephone-based service, and a partner from Children and Youth Services was there because he was very interested in the kind of linkages across children's families and the wider adults agenda, and we now know we need to think very carefully about how that links with an existing families information service and, you know, we hadn't directly made the connection but now it's yes actually, oh yes. So I think it can really help in making sure we're not duplicating and we're not reinventing wheels and we're building from the good stuff that's already happening ... locally." (Site 2)

Partnerships and Local Area Agreements

Respondents were asked to what extent the targets set out in their LAA impacted upon their own organisation and the partnership as a whole. The consensus view was that respondents acknowledged that their own targets contributed to the greater whole of the LAA target. Though conscious of the LAA target, organisations were, perhaps understandably, more focused on their own target as opposed to the LAA target as a whole. However, awareness of the LAA was present. Although not as predominant, the view was also expressed that the LAA targets set by the local authority were unattainable and unrealistic.

Public health partnerships: what are the benefits for service users?

As noted earlier, one of the main benefits of partnership working is through having a coordinated approach, whereby service users can be referred to the most appropriate agency with agencies acting in concert to provide clear referral pathways for users. Respondents were asked about the various advantages of, and difficulties associated with, such an approach and to give examples of how it operated to benefit service users. Given the nature of the four tracer issue study areas (smoking cessation, obesity, teenage pregnancy and alcohol reduction) and the number of agencies involved in the different aspects of these complex public health issues, referral pathways varied considerably. However, some common approaches could be discerned in referral pathways.

For smoking cessation in study site 3, referrals were commonly from GPs, pharmacies and health trainers in the locality and through self-referral by two stop smoking services based in the locality, one community-based and one business-based. In relation to study site 1 and alcohol reduction, users could be referred directly from hospital and, if fit, were either recommended to undertake a detoxification programme or given a choice of attending a clinic or receiving information about the dangers of over-consumption of alcohol. Users could also self-refer to a number of agencies helping with abstinence or alcohol reduction. There were also other pathways, for example, through the probation service. In study site 4 and teenage pregnancy, users could be referred from a GP, the education service, teenage pregnancy support youth workers or social services, for example, and a number of agencies in the area offered support for teenage mums and would-be teenage mums. In regard to obesity (site 2), referrals were either through GPs, dieticians, the advertising of various keep-fit activities or word of mouth.

We now consider respondents' views about the referral process and the advantages of working in partnership and how that benefits service users.

A more seamless service

As noted earlier, with agencies working together, a coordinated pathway could be offered to service users in order to ensure that they were referred to the most appropriate agency at the appropriate time. The following respondent gives an example of how this works in practice:

> "we get people coming through our door who need this service, that service, the other service, let's develop a system so that we can move our client ... from our service seamlessly into yours, so there is a continuum of care that can be tracked, that it's very clear who takes responsibility and when responsibility is handed over and that that is clear and it is understood what information passes between people and why.... So that's the big advantage, it's efficient and it's efficacious.... So the important thing is to make sure that you can move people through quickly and easily. So, you know, with identified pathways ... [it's] a bit like

going to the optician's, you get your eyes tested, 'Here's your prescription, take it where you want to get your glasses made up'. That's the obvious advantage. So what it does mean, of course, is that there is more money in the system because there is less duplication." (Executive Director, Alcohol Charity, site 1)

A smoking cessation advisor notes how working in partnership means being able to tackle a person's health problems, which may be multifaceted:

"it's no use someone coming to me, giving up smoking and then going, you know, 'I'm putting all this weight on, I'm sick of it', and you're going 'Oh that's awful that isn't it'. Whereas instead I'll say 'You know what, here's the information for the health trainers, they're absolutely brilliant', and [that's] what I'll do ... and then ... they don't get dumped out of the health and social care chain then. Once they leave [the smoking cessation service], they go and they join another health and social care chain, and they go around like that. And by keeping the client in the system that way with another agency, they're less likely to go back to smoking because they're taking a full lifestyle change; not just giving up smoking, they're doing it all in one go. So that works better I've found. I get more people [to] quit that way." (Site 3)

The difference partnership working makes to the lives of service users

Respondents were asked to give examples of how working in partnership aided service users. Apart from a more seamless service, and users being signposted to other services they may need, respondents identified a range of reasons to explain how partnerships made the service user experience a better one. Some examples of interviewees' accounts follow:

"I've had some success ... [when] working in partnership ... [it was] helping schools achieve healthy school status from a position a few years ago whereby we were sort of meeting government targets, but we were kind of only just meeting, to a point where we have now all our schools engaged on healthy school status; 98% of them are now through as healthy schools. That was only through partnership working between the authority and the schools or individuals from the schools that we ... got to that place." (Public Health Nutritionist, site 2)

"I think we can offer them a holistic service by being able to share. Because there's sometimes things I wouldn't be able to do alone, and I think having the benefit of like, for example, you know, I work with [another agency] very closely, and we sometimes do a lot of joint visiting between us, so I'll do my bit and ... [they] do their bit, and it's all in one visit if you like, so ... we put in place what we need to, and then obviously the following up and evaluating what we've done, you know, have we achieved what we set out to do, you know, have we got them rehoused, have we got them support, you know, have we sorted the contraception out, you know, they've got a healthy baby, they can access services. And I just think sometimes when you look at the outcomes and you've maybe helped support the partner and everybody else as well with benefits or jobs and things like that, I just think that is really sort of, you feel like you've done a good job if you like working together on something. And I think you can provide a lot, lot more for them by working together than being there on your own. You know, eventually, I mean, you'll probably get to the same outcome eventually possibly, but it can take a lot longer, whereas if you're actually sharing the load along the way with somebody, I think that young person benefits from that." (Specialist Midwife in Teenage Pregnancy, site 4)

Although working in partnership can offer a more seamless and holistic service, this is not always the case, as respondents did identify, as noted earlier, lack of information-sharing protocols, which could then entail service users being continually reassessed due to different assessment procedures being in place.

A not-so-seamless service

Respondents noted that although strides had been made to ensure that services were more coordinated and seamless for users, problems remained. Here, respondents give examples of service users who are constantly being reassessed:

> "hopefully, the patient is getting better treatment now and more choice. The only problem with that is, and this is the only guarded thing about partnership work, is that what we don't want to see is people having to jump through too many hoops. So that yeah, I want to self-refer, so I go to my GP. Now my GP hopefully would say go to ... our [service]. Now if I saw them and then said actually you look too heavyweight, you need to go to ... [another substance misuse service], you could be ... passed around from pillar to post a bit, which could be all right, but what we like to do with alcohol services is do assessments. And one of my bug bears is that we assess people to death." (Clinical Nurse Specialist, site 1)

> "in terms of, like, referral forms, we're all asking people to fill in the same information time and time and time again, whereas someone's had it to start with, so you could pass that information on to your partners to save the paperwork from the participants. I mean by the time you've done like two evaluation forms, two registers, it takes up a lot of your actual face-to-face contact time that you have with people, you think in that time you could have discussed another health message or another one of their concerns or reinforced something, but instead you're filling out [forms], and obviously you know we all need the paperwork, but do we all need our individual paperwork. I think that kind of thing can be frustrating for people I would imagine." (Community Health Development Officer, site 3)

The views of service users

Focus groups with service users in three of the four tracer issue areas (alcohol misuse, site 1; weight management, site 2; and teenage pregnancy, site 4) were conducted to ascertain their views on issues such as how well they felt services worked together and what improvements they perceived were needed, and their impressions of the service provision they had received.

How service users were referred to the service

The majority of users in regard to the weight management service were referred by their GP, or discovered the service through local advertising or word of mouth. For the alcohol misuse group, referrals were either through a GP, another provider or through self-referral. In regard to the teenage pregnancy focus group, referrals were generally from other agencies providing support and advice to (soon to be) teenage parents or through school.

Clear referral system to other providers

Focus group respondents were asked if there was clear help and advice for referral to other providers for any other issues they may need help with. Those in the weight management focus group were unclear about what help and advice was available, as these two respondents illustrate:

> "You see this is where we need to ... get everything together. Nobody knows what's going on, even the doctors don't refer you unless you ask them or somebody tells you." (Female, focus group, site 2)

> "What I found a bit, I suppose a bit disappointing, I was referred through my GP. I'm a diabetic so I have an annual check-up and my blood pressure was high and I take tablets for cholesterol, so my GP referred me, and my body mass index was very high. And my GP referred me and followed me, I used to go to the nurse but, of course, I don't know whether it's because when I went for my last annual check-up my blood pressure was down, my cholesterol was down etc.... I'm now left to get on with it myself. So that's one of the reasons that I've joined [the weight management group] as a premier club member so that I pay every month and I make sure I go. But the follow-up I'm a bit disappointed with, but I suppose that's life really." (Female, focus group, site 2)

Those in the alcohol focus group tended to be generally very aware of the services in their area and many of them had used a variety of them in the past, albeit with mixed views on their effectiveness and the referral process. However, this teenage male was a first-time user of the service and this was his experience:

"Well, I went to the GP at various times, because I've been living abroad and I came back and I was in a nervous state, and all the GP would say was 'You've got to cut your drinking back over a few days', which is really hard to take for someone who's, you know, if you're not being watched....But I didn't know anywhere to look or anything so I had my dad to thank for researching on the internet and pretty much driving me here in some sort of state, which I don't remember, but as everyone's said it's been quite helpful here." (Male, focus group, site 1)

How could services work more effectively together?

Service users had a variety of ideas concerning how services could work more effectively together and be more coordinated. As this female respondent notes, GPs need to be more proactive:

"I think GPs can do a lot more.... Most of us know our GPs or have a GP, and I think that if anyone has been there with any problem and they know that you're overweight or they know that you're smoking or whatever it is, then surely they should be trying to help you put that right. And they're the gateway to health, and I'm not sure they see it that way. And maybe it's become a sickness service, but I think that your practice nurses, your nurse practitioners, your GPs are key." (Female, focus group, site 2)

Generally, service users from the weight management focus group believed that services needed to be more joined-up and available through their local GP. The alcohol focus group also believed that GPs could do more to signpost and help service users, as this respondent makes clear:

"The GPs don't really give you any help because they don't know what they're talking about. You know, you can't just go to a GP and say 'Look, I need some help with this problem' because they haven't got a clue because they only have a grunt, you know, that they've never had a problem." (Male, focus group, site 1)

Of course, providing a joined-up and seamless service relies upon joined-up policy and procedures and strategic partnership working from service providers. Service providers believed that there were a number of policy and process issues that needed to be addressed to ensure more effective and joined-up service provision.

Service providers and policy process issues

Respondents voiced concerns in two areas of the policy process:

- a need for more strategic joined-up working between partners; and
- a disconnect between the top and bottom tiers of partnerships and within partner agencies.

Lack of strategic join-up

Partnerships sometimes suffered from a lack of strategic joined-up working, which prevented them from operating at their full potential. This deficit was voiced in a number of areas of partnership working, including the different legislative frameworks that agencies work within, which made achieving a cohesive and strategic partnership policy framework very difficult. The legislative frameworks of different agencies may be at cross purposes in some instances. Moreover, the plethora of strategies (ie alcohol and teenage pregnancy strategies) needed bringing together into an aligned and coherent whole. The overall impression is that strategic join-up is still far from being realised. This respondent gives an example of the lack of cohesiveness as experienced by them:

> "what the council have done, slightly bizarrely, again shows probably not high-enough-level people being involved, is that their corporate directors have ... recently decided they were going to have a meeting about alcohol ... and my Director of Public Health got to hear at the last minute. They were basically, some council person was asked to pull out all the stuff that other people are doing elsewhere and then look at what we were doing, which felt totally bizarre. We've got all these people working on alcohol already, and suddenly these people who didn't know anything about it suddenly coming along and deciding they're going to make all these suggestions. So I did have an ability to influence some of the content at the last minute ... my frustration was that none of us who are working all the time know and weren't told about it, weren't involved until suddenly at the

last minute someone came along. Oh goodness, it was too late to change much." (Public Health Consultant, site 1)

A Specialist Midwife in Teenage Pregnancy acknowledges the gaps in bringing various public health strands together into a coherent whole:

"I think we can acknowledge that they need to be linked. I think we're actually acknowledging that they're the same, you know, the same themes are coming through, and I think it took us a long time to see that, and I think it's been about oh we do alcohol here, we do this, there and that, and we've not sort of noticed along the way that all of those have an impact on everybody else. So I do think we are getting better but I do think it has been poor in the past, and I think it's been very isolated, you know, we go off and we do the alcohol strategy, we go off and do the teenage pregnancy strategy. Whereas I think now we're getting to realise, as that board, as a group, that it affects, it has an impact on everything, you know, each individual service has got the same issues if you like. You know, the individuals that we're [coming] across have got the same issues." (Site 4)

As above, so below?

There was a general consensus that partnerships tended to operate more effectively from a bottom-up perspective than from a top-down one. There was evidence of some disconnect between the top of some partner organisations and the front line in these same organisations. Three respondents encapsulate these themes:

"I've had some experiences where people at a senior level pay lip service to it [partnership], whereas the people on the ground are very engaged with the concept, but at the senior level, it's not." (Tobacco Control Commissioner, site 3)

"my experience is actually that one of the good things about grassroot clinicians and workers is that they naturally form partnerships just by written protocols or service level agreements that are mutually beneficial and are most often very, very client-centred. And I think when you start to look at wider partnerships and trying to pin that down on paper, it's very easy to overlook those individual flexible relationships that have existed for a long, long time." (Dual Diagnosis Clinical Director, site 1)

"I mean, there are some people in organisations that are signed up at the strategic level who simply will not play, and they seem to get away with it, which is beyond my understanding but that's it ... there's a lot of tokenism, a lot of tokenism. But the reality is that it's the front-line workers that make a difference, you know." (Executive Director, Alcohol Charity, site 1)

Capacity, commissioning and competition

Lack of capacity of the voluntary sector

This issue, while not a major theme and not an issue put directly to participants, was highlighted by Directors of Public Health, Directors of Commissioning and other senior managers as an issue in the earlier phase of the research, reported in Chapter Four, and was highlighted again in this phase. There were concerns over whether the voluntary sector had the necessary capacity to tender for services, together with a concern from the voluntary sector over the short timescales for bidding for contracts. Two respondents highlight some of these issues:

"You can sometimes get very short timescales for the pieces of work they're commissioning in order to get a bid in, and actually incredibly short timescales to deliver them in as well, and, of course, there may be kind of national organisations that will do a piece of, sort of attitude research for you at the drop of a hat, but if you actually want to engage somebody locally to do it, you know, their timescales are absolutely potty and then they do nothing with the information for a year, and you think 'Okay, we've just killed ourselves trying to deliver that for you within two months when it could have been done over three or four and then you did nothing with the information for a year' – it's hugely frustrating." (Environmental Charity Manager, site 2)

"to have a thriving local and third sector ... we're all committed to that, and it's very frustrating for us to be able to have to give money to the statutory sector or to one of the bigger ... and larger third sector organisations ...

who seem to win most of the money. But when we apply the procurement law, it's very difficult not to do that, even though we're sort of rooting mostly on the local bid. You know, in terms of law and the challenge and risk, you're almost now forced to take on the big boys, and we would rather be utilising some of our local providers. And we just reorganised our drug treatment centres, so it's a fundamental whole-system change, and it's going to be an enormous amount of procurement and new projects over the next three years, and we've involved our local voluntary sector in that, and we're encouraging them. We've had events with the national providers to introduce them to the local providers so they can work together. But that's all we can do. We can't create a situation where we say 'We're going to give this to a local provider'." (Director of Strategy and Commissioning, Alcohol Partnership, site 1)

Competition and partnerships

Concerns were raised about the collaborative nature of partnership working on the one hand, with many of its central features (as we have noted) being based on goodwill and trust, and the active encouragement being given to competition and market-testing among prospective providers on the other. The view expressed was that the competitive nature of agencies competing for funding under the NHS commissioning process risked clashing with the partnership ethos, thereby giving rise to tensions within the partnership. There was also some concern over partners 'talking up' how well their service was performing to other partners for fear of being decommissioned. Such issues take on an added significance in the context of the Coalition government's health and social care reforms, introduced in 2013, which have at their heart a focus on competition and choice as the principal means to drive up quality, promote innovation and offer a more cost-effective and productive service (see Chapter Six). From our study, the following three respondents illustrate these points:

"It can affect relationships when ... the authority commissions out to an organisation that's already around locally, and another loses out there, that could definitely create a problem." (Public Health Nutritionist, site 2) "and I think that's one of the things that we notice in a sense, that with one provider we suggested that we, because we're such a small service and we have limited resources, we suggested that actually we could do joint training, and they were very reluctant to do that because basically we were talking about two competitors getting in the same room together. So that was a bit disingenuous in a way. But, equally, they have to work together as well and they have to form their own partnerships. So I think that can fracture partnerships a little bit." (Dual Diagnosis Clinical Director, site 1)

"I mean there is a problem with people being honest about waiting times. Because the more partners you've got round the table, the same amount of money, and so ... everyone's got to be savvy about saying how well the service is doing. That's one of my bug bears of partnership working is that you hear from clients or you hear from other partners around the table that things aren't going so well at a service, but then when you are around the table, everything's very rosy and there's not a problem. And I find that very difficult to deal with because I see why it happens, because obviously you don't want your service to be decommissioned, but it's not necessarily helpful when you hear that 'Oh, my waiting time is only three weeks' when actually you've just referred someone who knows it's about six. And that can be a problem with the partnership working; the more partners, the less money." (Clinical Nurse Specialist, site 1)

The bottom line – do the benefits of partnerships outweigh the costs?

Given that partnerships are not cost-free and they incur significant resource costs, respondents were asked whether they felt that partnerships could justify these costs in terms of the outcomes gained. The consensus was that partnerships could be justified since the benefits they bestowed far outweighed the costs incurred. However, a minority of respondents were a little more circumspect on the issue.

Of those who gave an unqualified 'yes' to this question, there were a myriad of responses as to why. Among these were that partnerships were more cost-efficient because of economies of scale (ie the costs were shared between partners and the return was greater because of the number of agencies contributing to the outcome). Less duplication and more efficient targeting of resources through a coordinated approach were other factors cited. There were also the intangible assets, such as the costs saved from individuals quitting smoking or drinking, or taking part in healthy eating and exercise regimes, and the savings realised in respect of easing future demand on the NHS and wider society. These respondents highlight some of these themes:

> "The answer is yes, because what you don't do necessarily in these cost–benefit analyses is look at the longevity of the savings that you make on that individual by them not being in care and not being in prison, not ... [needing] medical attention and so on and so forth. So I think we have to be really, really careful with some of these projects where they might look that the partnership working and the human and financial resources that have gone into it look to be huge, that we don't purely do a cost–benefit analysis on what's happening today." (Leisure and Culture Development Manager, site 2)

> "Most definitely, in terms of, well, for every two people I see, I save a life, as they say. The cost of NHS care for the people with the likes of COPD [Chronic Obstructive Pulmonary Disease] and, you know, the treatment of lung cancer, etc, yeah, [its] a high cost-effective way ... [for] Health, most definitely." (Health Protection Advisor, site 3)

Of those who were a little more circumspect about the issue of whether or not partnerships justified their cost, the view was expressed that until tangible outcomes were proved to exist as a result of the partnership, the jury was still out. Since lots of intangible assets of partnership working could not be factored into a precise calculation of costs and benefits, it was difficult to give a clear and unequivocal judgement about cause and effect. There was also the view that partnerships performed well in some areas but perhaps not so well in others. A Lead Clinician Team Leader states:

> "it's a bit like the old WHO [World Health Organization] vaccination policy for smallpox some years ago. I remember reading a paper on it and somebody asked a very neat question which was: 'Does the smallpox vaccination policy work?' Well, two questions about it. One is if it works, why

are we still doing it? And if it doesn't work, why are we still doing it? And I think it's the same with this, because if it still needs holding together, in other words, if somebody wasn't still putting a lot of energy and investment into holding it, why are we still needing to hold it? Why hasn't it come together? Why is it still continuing to apparently pull in opposite directions? And I think that answers the question because if they're not coming together after the length of time of being together, maybe they're so disparate that they shouldn't be together in that format." (Site 1)

Discussion – partnerships at the front line: what works and what does not?

For those working on the front line, partnerships have much to commend themselves. Working in partnership was not only regarded as providing a coordinated approach to tackling public health issues, but also viewed as being of major benefit to service users by giving them a more seamless service and acting as a signpost for other services they may need to access. Different agency perspectives, it was believed, could lead to innovative solutions in tackling public health issues. Through utilising the shared knowledge and expertise of partner agencies, this meant that service users could benefit by having access to a variety of services on a number of levels, from access to a youth worker to help with finding a home.

Sharing information and having established information–sharing protocols again ensured that service users did not always have to give the same information to all other services with which they came into contact. However, a finding from the research is that this remains work in progress and there are still instances of poor information sharing and a lack of sharing protocols between agencies.

It is clear, too, that networking was very important, both for those working at the front line and at a middle management level. Networking brought the prospect of further collaborative work with other agencies and could potentially aid the coordinated approach of service delivery, with partners being aware of the latest developments in practice nationally and locally. It also gave agencies the opportunity to see where their policies and priorities aligned and to shape their policies and practices towards collaborative working accordingly.

Goodwill between agencies was regarded very much as the glue that holds partnerships together, particularly on the front line. It was also the case that 'local champions' played a crucial role in networks, acting as conduits for sharing information. However, given the length of time partnerships have been in operation, it is perhaps only to be expected that they are now perceived as the natural, if not the only, way of doing things. Arguably, with policy and procedures firmly embedded, perhaps there should not be so much reliance on something as fragile and ephemeral as goodwill in order for partnerships to function.

Organisational change can be very disruptive to partnership networks, with partnerships having to be reconstituted because of such turbulence. What this says about the destructive and destabilising influence of organisational change on the one hand, or the enduring strength of partnerships on the other, is open to debate.

Different agency perspectives are an issue and can negate, or limit the potential of, effective partnerships. By this, we mean that an agency's own statutory priorities and targets invariably take precedence over their obligations to the partnership. This begs the question of how far joint partnership targets should become more commonplace in order to encourage and cement the partnership approach, instead of there being targets and priorities for individual organisations that are likely to take precedence and pull organisations in opposite directions.

It was found that not all partner organisations were aware of their respective roles and responsibilities within the partnership. Once again, this raises questions concerning partnerships' methods of accountability and their effectiveness, in addition to the leverage they can exert to hold individual agencies to account.

Service users voiced their concern that GPs, for example, were not acting as a gateway to refer users to services that were available in their particular locality. Users were frustrated by the fact that a range of services could be available in their community of which they had no knowledge. They were obliged to make requests to agency providers to discover such information. Yet, practitioners cited partnership working as the vehicle for providing a seamless service and acting as a signpost to refer users to other services if required. It is clear that service users did not see this happening in practice and the lack of information as to what services were available in their communities was a significant source of frustration. There seems to be a clear disconnect here between what level of service practitioners think they are providing and the actual experience of service provision by users. Perhaps partner agencies would benefit from making an effort to discover user knowledge of the services being offered in their locality, with a view, if necessary, to rectifying any knowledge gaps.

It was noted that there was a lack of horizontal and vertical strategic join-up in partnerships. Different areas of public health policy were not aligned to provide a cohesive framework (ie the teenage pregnancy strategy not being aligned with the alcohol strategy in one of the study sites). There were also concerns over the apparent gulf between front-line practitioners and senior management. The partnership approach on the front line appeared to be a more organic and holistic process, with partnerships formed clearly and flexibly with the desire to deliver a more coordinated experience for service users. This contrasted with senior management approaches, where the emphasis was firmly on a target-setting ethos to deliver on key themes. The consensus among practitioners was that partnerships that worked effectively were essentially 'bottom-up' in origin rather than 'top-down', with partnerships forged from the bottom up being based around delivering on the needs of service users and constructed from practical necessity and direct experience of what was required.

Although not directly addressed in the study, it was believed that, in some instances, the smaller voluntary sector agencies did not have the capacity to deliver services. Concern was also expressed over the competitive element of bidding for commissioned services and how this could fracture the collaborative approach of partnerships and potentially sour relations between agencies. Moreover, as we seek to show in Chapter Six, in the new competitive environment being actively developed in the NHS following the passage of the Health and Social Care Act 2012, smaller third sector organisations are unable to compete on the same basis as larger private sector providers, which are geared up for the task. Many are therefore having their funding cut and find themselves unable to compete on a level playing field.

Finally, there was a strongly held belief that the financial and human resource costs invested in partnership working were worthwhile in terms of the outcomes gained and that agencies were obliged to work in partnership because no single agency could on its own deliver the range of services or possess all the expertise to deliver on such complex public health issues. Despite this, it remained difficult to pinpoint how outcomes had been directly influenced or determined by partnership working, thereby reaffirming the view that a great deal of faith in it persists.

Despite respondents' belief that partnership working is the most appropriate mechanism to deliver complex public health goals, issues such as differing priorities among agencies, each with its own targets to deliver at the expense and neglect of the partnership, combined with such issues as lack of information sharing and lack of clarity over roles and responsibilities in partnerships, show that tensions and countervailing pressures can work against partnerships. For all the rhetoric surrounding them, and claims made for them, some fundamental core issues remain to be addressed if partnerships are to function more effectively in the future for the benefit of the populations they exist to serve.

Conclusion: from top to bottom – lessons to be learned about partnership working

With the study focusing on those responsible for shaping and planning public health objectives, as well as on front-line practitioners tasked with implementing and delivering these objectives, while also obtaining the views of service users in receipt of such services, a number of key themes from those working at the strategic management level and at the front line can be discerned.

A successful public health partnership is one that recognises that partnership working needs to be embedded in the culture from the bottom to the top in each partner organisation and between agencies. The partnership needs to be clear and realistic about its goals, adaptive and flexible, and needs to avoid too heavy an emphasis on structures; instead, it needs to be more holistic and organic in its approach to tackling 'wicked issues' in public health, paying particular attention to relational issues. This means being innovative and flexible and perhaps showing a willingness to take risks.

Our research found that, in practice:

- Those partnerships deemed to be successful in their own terms were those in which the policy processes were outcomes-focused, with joint delivery mechanisms, clear lines of accountability, the full engagement of relevant partners and careful monitoring in place. Conversely, less successful partnerships were deemed to be deficient in respect of many or all of these key features. But any policy goals or targets need to be owned by partner agencies from top to bottom and there need to be 'policy threads' that link organisations both vertically and horizontally. Crucially, those working at the front line should not be subject to 'terror by targets', but listened to and actively encouraged to discuss what works and how those at a more senior level can facilitate an approach that has the service users at its core in creating a more seamless service and not so much a target-driven approach. This seems to be the chief lesson to emerge from the Francis inquiry into the serious and appalling lapses in patient care that occurred at the Mid Staffordshire Hospitals Foundation Trust over a period of four years between 2005 and 2009 despite concerns raised repeatedly by patients and carers (Francis, 2013). Logic would dictate that if the public health needs of service users are met, then this would achieve the target(s) to be delivered. At the present time, the approach is more akin to putting the cart before the horse (target first and service users second, or possibly third).

- Sharing information between agencies and having established information-sharing protocols avoided duplication and encouraged a coordinated approach. This was found to be the case among front-line practitioners and those at a strategic level.

- An effective partnership was where all the agencies involved were aware of their respective roles and responsibilities – again, a lesson learned regardless of where an employee was located in the hierarchical structure.

- A good partnership focused upon the needs of service users, ensuring that they did not always have to give the same information to every other service with which they came into contact in the public health and related arenas. The major benefit to service users, apart from a more seamless service, was acting as a signpost for other services they may need to access. Unfortunately, the needs of service users and how a coordinated approach can greatly benefit them seemed to get somewhat lost at the strategic level, where the emphasis was almost exclusively on targets, strategic plans and policy and procedures.

- Goodwill and trust between agencies was seen very much as the glue that holds partnerships together, particularly on the front line, but also among senior practitioners. It was also the case that 'local champions' played a crucial role in partnerships and they should be nurtured and supported at all levels.

- Different agency perspectives, it was believed, could lead to innovative solutions in tackling public health issues, from policy formulation to practical everyday contexts, by sharing knowledge and the expertise of the various partner agencies.

- A successful partnership is marked by pragmatism, flexibility and an organic quality, which gets lost at higher levels, where the approach adopted is much more formal and mechanistic, governed by which structures are required to be put in place and which targets are to be met. The former qualities were very much in evidence with partnerships formed at the front line, which were much more flexible, holistic and organic in their approach to tackling public health issues and, as a result, were deemed more successful in pursuing their stated goals.

At the other extreme, the message from many of our respondents at all levels is that partnerships that are failing to deliver suffer from a number of common elements, namely:

• a lack of good information-sharing protocols in place;

• partners not being clear about their roles and responsibilities;

• a failure to ensure that targets are shared and owned by the partnership so that agencies do not disengage when their own targets and priorities become pressing;

• targets can induce a silo mentality, hence the need for shared partnership targets;

• front-line practitioners generally held the view that partnerships operate best from the bottom up when they are formed to address the needs of service users in the hope of offering a more coordinated service with less duplication and clear pathways for referral. Such partnerships were seen as more organic and holistic, relying on sharing information, good networking and information-sharing protocols that were agreed pragmatically and flexibly as needs arose;

• there appears to be a disconnect from the top to the bottom in some partnerships, where information does not flow easily from the top down and the communication of goals and priorities is not clear or consistent. In addition, a sense of common ownership of targets and priorities is not evident in all cases, with clear communication, sharing of information and engagement at all levels of the partnership being regarded as essential prerequisites of high trust relationships; and

• it remains the case that too much emphasis is placed on policy processes and structures and not enough on outcomes. A more outcomes-based approach seems desirable, with lessons to be learned from front-line practitioners who may have developed solutions based on particular service users' needs in a holistic and streamlined manner, rather than through complex policy processes that, as we have noted, can take the focus away from an outcomes-based approach.

Although partnership working received positive support in the main from our study sites and those we interviewed, digging a little deeper into its processes and structures revealed a more nuanced picture, which begins to question the need for some of the existing, and often elaborate, partnership structures. They may endeavour to be all-inclusive but can at the same time become unwieldy, overly complex and cumbersome. Therefore, the need for more loosely based partnerships as a way of doing business, derived from sound relationships and formed to perform certain functions and tasks, which are then disbanded when these goals have been accomplished, may merit further consideration along the lines suggested in Chapter Two.

SIX

The changing policy context: new dawn or poisoned chalice?

Over the period covered by this book, between the late 1990s and 2012, health policy has been in a state of perpetual change. This is less true elsewhere in the UK than in England, where there has been a rapid succession of policy and organisational changes, initially under the Labour government (1997–2010) and then under the Coalition government (from 2010 to the present). In the other countries making up the UK, with the arrival of devolution at the close of the 1990s, the three countries (Wales, Scotland and Northern Ireland) have adopted different models and a different pace of change (for up-to-date reviews of health policy in each of the four UK countries see the 'Health systems in transition' reports from the European Observatory on Health Systems and Policies, Boyle, 2011; Longley et al, 2012; O'Neill et al, 2012; Steel and Cylus, 2012).

With the election of what turned out to be a Coalition government in May 2010, there was no expectation of major change in the health sector, as the Prime Minister, David Cameron, had publicly and explicitly ruled out further 'top-down' reorganisation of the NHS on the grounds that there had been quite enough of it already, much of which had failed to achieve its intended objectives. The Coalition agreement mentioned making Primary Care Trusts more democratic but there was no suggestion of a major wholesale restructuring affecting virtually every part of the NHS and public health. Nor did the government have a mandate from the electorate for major change since none had been proposed or considered during the election campaign. But it seems that the then Secretary of State for Health, Andrew Lansley, had different ideas and had in fact a plan for significant change in an advanced stage of readiness in the event that he would be in a position to unveil it and put it into operation.

Two White Papers published in 2012 set the scene for arguably the biggest change agenda in the history of both the NHS and public health (Hunter, 2011). The NHS White Paper was published in July 2010, barely two months after entering office (Secretary of State for Health, 2010a), with the public health White Paper following six months or so later (Secretary of State for Health, 2010b). Yet again, all those working in the NHS (or rather all those able, or prepared, to remain) were about to embark on what the NHS chief executive, David Nicholson, termed 'a journey of change'. Few could understand why such a journey was needed or was being pursued with such vigour in the face of major reservations about aspects of Lansley's grand plan. While the direction of travel was broadly consistent with New Labour's NHS reforms, the Coalition government clearly wanted to go much further and faster, with the result that little of the NHS was left untouched by the proposed changes. It was the sheer scale of the changes that caused the NHS chief executive to quip that they were so big that they could be seen from space.

The changes were presented as putting both patients and GPs at the centre of decision-making and resource allocation so that care and services would be responsive to local needs and circumstances. Indeed, localism was a theme of much of the government's policymaking when it came to public services and the future role of the state in their provision. But, as in other areas of public policy, the changes were also designed to open up the NHS to greater competition and marketisation, although these aspects of the changes were played down by the government. The commodification of health care, begun under New Labour, was to be rolled out with even greater enthusiasm and urgency against the backdrop of the nation's financial deficit, which had to be tackled, so the government asserted, through a substantial programme of public spending cuts. Finally, the changes were intended to reduce bureaucracy and costs by stripping out layers of management that would no longer be necessary in a service driven by local concerns rather than steered by the centre.

In fact, following a series of modifications to the original proposals to accommodate numerous concerns, the end result is a structure that is far more complex than that originally proposed and with several new layers of management added to replace those that have been removed. The overall financial cost of the changes is likely to far exceed any savings and is entirely in keeping with the available evidence, as a review of central government reorganisations from the National Audit Office (NAO) revealed (National Audit Office, 2010a). The NAO reported more than 90 reorganisations to British central government over a four-year period from May 2005 to June 2009 and put the cost of each reorganisation as at approximately £200 million per annum. Separately, Walshe (2010) estimated the cost of the proposed NHS changes at £2–£3 billion to implement at a time of severe financial austerity and when the NHS was being required to save £20 billion by 2014.

All the proposed NHS changes met with near-universal opposition from the professional bodies and groups representing the public. The public health proposals were generally received with a warmer welcome, although there were a few critics, especially those from a clinical background who had pursued an NHS career in public health (McKee et al, 2011). In respect of the changes overall, the media and public were for the most part simply baffled and mistakenly viewed them, or were encouraged to view them, as principally technocratic in nature rather than as an assault on the founding principles of the NHS and public health care, which critics of the proposals alleged. Opposition to the changes from professional groups tended to be dismissed by many in the media and by some members of the public as the product of special pleading – a misconceived attempt to protect outmoded perks and privileges.

But the media, and those sections of the public that subscribed to this view, could not have been more mistaken, since underlying the changes was a very clear and explicit political philosophy and one that had been articulated by some Conservatives well before the election. As two seasoned academic observers of the political scene put it:

> the coalition programme is more than an immediate response to a large current account deficit. It involves a restructuring of welfare benefits and public services that takes the country in a new direction, rolling back the state to a level of intervention below that in the United States – something which is unprecedented....The policies include substantial privatisation and a shift of responsibility from state to individual. (Taylor-Gooby and Stoker, 2011, p 14)

Against this febrile and fractured context to the government's unpopular NHS and public health changes, this chapter offers an overview of the key changes enshrined in the Health and Social Care Act 2012 as far as they impact on public health and the future of partnership working. The changes affecting public health, in particular, carry with them major implications for the future of partnerships. For some engaged in public health policy and practice, they herald an exciting new opportunity to learn the lessons from past failed or poorly performing partnerships in order to put in place a new approach that merely tinkering with previous arrangements would not have achieved. But for others, the upheaval can only result in the loss from public health of valuable networks, relationships and expertise, with the consequence that new partnerships will have to be formed all over again and the risk that old mistakes are merely repeated. They argue that the upheaval will result in a loss of progress and momentum, will incur significant costs as new partnerships are formed, and could result in minimal impact in respect of improved outcomes as the new organisations will inevitably lack maturity and will take time to deliver any promised improvements. The fact that all of this is occurring at a time when the NHS is undergoing major change throughout its structure and when the public sector generally, especially local government, is being subjected to an unprecedented, though quite deliberate, squeeze on public finances can only exacerbate the problems and make partnership working more difficult as groups and organisations are disbanded and reformed in new configurations.

So, while the glass appears half-full for some, for others, it is half-empty. But it remains too soon to pass judgement on whether the optimists or pessimists are right. Those in either camp can point to particular developments and features to support their position. Take as an example the finding from a survey of Directors of Public Health (DsPH) conducted by the Association of DsPH in 2012, which suggested that two thirds of current DsPH were either looking to leave employment or seek it in the NHS somewhere rather than have to transfer to local government. Although the news caused panic in some quarters, in others, the ostensible 'crisis' about to befall the public health workforce offered an opportunity to break out of the prevailing professional mind traps and do things differently. After all, it is argued, if you want real change, especially that involving culture and behaviour, then it makes little sense to adopt a policy of 'lift and shift' if, by doing so, the old guard are allowed to lead the change, since the chances are that a situation of 'more of the same' will prevail.

The new health policy landscape

The changes being implemented across the NHS and public health, which came into effect in April 2013, entail new structures, some of which were operating in shadow form since 2012, if not earlier. While the new NHS arrangements will continue to have some public health functions, the lead for public health locally now lies with local government and nationally with a new body, Public Health England (PHE). We briefly consider the key NHS changes first before turning to public health, where we explore the changes in greater detail.

The NHS

First, to shift decision-making closer to patients, power and responsibility for commissioning services is being transferred to Clinical Commissioning Groups (CCGs), ostensibly led by GPs. Some 212 of these new bodies have replaced the former 152 Primary Care Trusts and 10 Strategic Health Authorities. Second, to support the new CCGs, another piece of structural apparatus has been created, initially called the NHS Commissioning Board (NHSCB), later to become known as NHS England. Based in Leeds, it is independent from ministers and the Department of Health, although it operates within a mandate from the Secretary of State for Health (Department of Health, 2012a). The first mandate will cover a two-year period from April 2013 to March 2015. Billed as 'the first of its kind in the world', it plays 'a vital role in setting out the strategic direction' for the NHS in England and ensuring that it remains properly accountable (Department of Health, 2012a, pp 4–5). It is the principal basis of ministerial instruction to the NHS, which will be 'operationally independent and clinically-led' (Department of Health, 2012a, p 5). The mandate cannot be changed in the course of the year without the agreement of the Board of NHS England. In turn, the Board is required to implement the objectives set out in the mandate. Rather optimistically, given that the new structures will require time to bed down, the mandate insists that if the Board is successful, then by March 2015, 'improvement across the NHS will be clear'. Of course, this timing is politically critical in that a general election can be held no later than May 2015 and the government will be seeking to showcase NHS improvements when the campaigning for re-election commences.

The mandate sets out the key objectives identified as being of greatest importance to the public. One concerns public health and the prevention of ill-health and premature death. Part of the objective here is to work with PHE (see later) to support local government in the roll-out of NHS health checks, for which local authorities became responsible after April 2013.

On a day-to-day basis, so the theory goes, ministers will not be able to interfere with the workings of NHS England and it is the NHS chief executive who will become the NHS's public face. From previous failed attempts in the 1990s to separate the operational workings of the NHS from its strategic direction, making the new arrangements work in practice will not be easy and ministers will find it difficult not to intervene if problems arise and become headlines in the media.

NHS England will provide leadership for quality improvement through commissioning and will distribute the budget to CCGs (some 60% of the total) while top-slicing funds for specialised services. If CCGs are not up to scratch or fail, NHS England can step in to run services directly or bring in new management. Although the government has sought to remove the regional tier from the NHS, NHS England operates sub-nationally through four regions, with 27 local area teams functioning below this level.

However, there are two particular problems with the NHS changes that have dogged them from the outset. First, few GPs actually want to spend their time on commissioning services and even fewer have the requisite skills for the task. To be able to commission effectively for a whole population requires a scale of activity that probably demands larger and fewer CCGs and certainly a different mindset among the majority of GPs. But, of course, the trade-off is that if CCGs get larger, then they cease to be local and close to their patients and local communities. It is a conundrum that has bedevilled commissioning, regardless of its precise configuration, since its inception in the early 1990s under the GP fundholding scheme.

Second, the changes are designed to promote choice and competition and to encourage market forces under the mantra of 'any qualified provider' to stimulate innovation and drive up quality and efficiency. The evidence for such a policy is scant and what exists is fiercely contested (Cooper et al, 2011; Gaynor et al, 2012; Pollock et al, 2011). However, it is not evidence but, as we have suggested, ideology that is the chief factor behind the policy. The Coalition government's primary purpose is to reduce public spending and to open up monopoly public services like health and education to private (both for-profit and not-for-profit) providers. But while competition is a key theme of the changes, so is the notion of integration and a desire to achieve better integrated care between all sectors of the health system – public health, primary care, secondary care and social care. With an ageing population and growing pressures on the NHS coming from non-communicable diseases, together with the possibility to treat many conditions outside hospital, the focus on care pathways and integration has come to the fore as a government priority. Indeed, Jeremy Hunt, who replaced Lansley as the Secretary of State for Health in 2012, and his team of ministers have placed the topic high on the policy agenda. What is at stake, however, is whether it is possible to have both competition and collaboration or whether it is necessary to sacrifice, or strictly limit, one to achieve the other. Many observers consider that it is not possible to have both and that the fracturing of care among a plurality of providers, many of them driven by profit and the need to maximise shareholder value and unaccountable to local communities, puts at risk an ethos of working collaboratively in an integrated fashion and being held to account for what happens.

Of course, as our own research into partnerships (described in Chapters Four and Five) has shown, even within a system where services are publicly funded and provided, there is no guarantee that integration and effective partnership working will be achieved. Such issues go deeper and derive from culture, the nature of professionalism and notions of leadership. All of these can and do have a profound effect on whether services work effectively together or at cross purposes. Nevertheless, there is concern among practitioners that the latest changes will threaten already well-run services and that if chunks of, say, community services are put out to tender and run by a different, and possibly a for-profit, provider, then there is a serious risk of breakdown both in continuity along the care pathway, or patient journey, and consistency of purpose. There is also an issue about accountability, especially when private companies are looking to secure shareholder value and these shareholders may reside many thousands of miles away in another country, if not continent.

Such developments are unlikely to impact on public health directly, although even here there are tensions between how best to tackle the problems of childhood obesity, sexual health and alcohol misuse – is it by taking on the powerful food and drinks companies through imposing tough regulation (smoking being a case in point) on them, or is it by agreeing responsibility deals of the kind favoured by some in the Coalition government, which involve working with the food and drinks industries and making progress through voluntary agreements? At present, policy seems to be rather confused and reactive and swings between the two, as in respect of (the now seemingly ill-fated) proposals for the minimum pricing for alcohol, which cuts across the responsibility deal policy in England.

Like the NHS, public health policy since 2010 has been largely dominated by significant restructuring. It is to the changes arising from this that we now turn, with a focus on what they might mean for partnership working.

Public health

The changes to public health are among the most interesting and unexpected. As in the case of the NHS changes, they were not mentioned in the run-up to the May 2010 general election. Yet, they are every bit as significant, and arguably more so, since they herald a return of the public health function to local government, from whence it was removed in 1974 at the time of the first major NHS reorganisation.

The public health reform marks a dramatic departure, in contrast to the NHS changes, which largely continue down the road, if more rapidly and on a grander scale, already embarked upon under the former Labour government. And the policy landscape and public health challenges are rather different from what they were back in the 1970s when public health came under local government control. This is recognised in the government's wish to return public health to local government while making it clear that the move is not about recreating a pre-1974 landscape. It is an acknowledgement of the fact that, in recent years, local government has taken on 'a much wider role of shaping local places. Having taken on the key role in promoting economic, social and environmental wellbeing at the local level, it is ideally placed to adopt a wider wellbeing role' (Department of Health, 2011a). In so doing, local authorities will have to work with a wide range of partners across civil society and the chief mechanism for this will be the leadership of Health and Wellbeing Boards (HWBs), which we consider later.

Some of the public health functions transferred to local government are mandatory. These include: providing appropriate access to sexual health services; ensuring that there are plans in place to protect the population's health, including immunisation and screening plans; ensuring that NHS commissioners receive public health advice on matters such as health needs assessments for particular conditions or disease groups and advice on a range of matters known as the 'core offer' from public health to CCGs; the NHS health check programme for people aged between 40 and 74; activities relating to the schools medical programme (eg duties to weigh and measure school children), including the transfer of the whole of the school nursing service, that is, those nurses who work in a public health role with school-aged children and their families (an exception here for a time at least is children aged 0–5 years, for whom NHS England will be responsible for their public health until 2015, when it is proposed that the responsibility be transferred to local authorities); and support for public health in prisons.

It is perhaps worth noting that the role of local government in public health, including tackling the social determinants of health, is increasingly recognised in many other European countries, as a report published by the World Health Organization (WHO) Regional Office for Europe emanating from the work of Marmot and his team on inequalities for health undertaken for WHO both globally and within

Europe demonstrates (Grady and Goldblatt, 2012). There are two key reasons for this development: because health is viewed as largely being socially determined; and to stimulate change by reducing central influence and promoting local autonomy, for which the structures underpinning local government are particularly well-suited. It is argued that greater local autonomy may lead to more flexible and efficient policies as local authorities are closer to their communities and able to respond more quickly to address their needs (Litvack et al, 1998). Furthermore, the WHO report claims that in a recession, the role of local government becomes even more important, 'especially in cities and urban areas, with a vital role to play in fostering and enhancing local health, well-being and resilience' (Grady and Goldblatt, 2012, p 2). The place-shaping role of local authorities is especially important and develops a theme that lay at the heart of the Lyons inquiry into the purpose of local government in England in the 21st century (Lyons, 2007).

The WHO report identified six implementation factors of particular importance. The following four factors are especially critical in the context of partnership working and all featured prominently in the research we reported on in the last two chapters:

- multiagency, multidisciplinary partnerships and collaboration;
- policy alignment and convergence;
- developing capability and capacity; and
- managing the political environment.

The first point in this list constitutes a particular implementation challenge facing local government across the European countries studied. It involves building and strengthening the leadership role of local government, especially working across sectors, and coordinating initiatives. The issue is compounded by the existence of complex partnership arrangements combined with the complexity of multiple agendas and perspectives, which makes reaching agreement difficult. The study also found 'that multiple departments or actors are often working on the same subject, almost working in the same way, but are still not cooperating' (Grady and Goldblatt, 2012, p 38). The issue of policy alignment and coherence is also of critical importance. It has always been a problem in terms of central–local relations across the NHS and local government and is likely to become even more pressing given the new structures being established both nationally and locally. We consider these later in this chapter.

Returning to the changes proposed for public health in England, chief among these has been the relocation of DsPH and their teams. Since April 2013, they have been transferred to local government from the NHS, where they were located in 1974. Although the introduction of joint posts over the past 10 years or so has resulted in some DsPH spending more time in, and looking out towards, local government, their success has been patchy. The return of the function to local government is a major structural and cultural change because DsPH will become employees of local government and be accountable to elected members for the discharge of their responsibilities. However, it is a little more complicated than this because the DsPH will also be accountable to the Secretary of State for Health in central government for certain functions, notably, in the area of health protection and emergency preparedness. Any dismissal of a DPH will require the minister's approval.

The arrangement is less than ideal from a local government perspective since it is unprecedented for a local government officer to be jointly accountable to a government minister. However, the Local Government Association did win an important concession in that the Secretary of State does not have the power to terminate the employment of a DPH, although it was an option in initial proposals. The local authority as the employer does have this power but it must consult the Secretary of State before exercising it. As lead advisor on health to the local authority and a statutory chief officer, the DPH will be an important official, influencing decisions across the whole range of an authority's business. The expectation is that there will be direct accountability between the DPH and local authority chief executive, although it can also be through another head of paid service. In practice, most local authorities have followed this advice and their DsPH are accountable to the chief executive. But in a few places, the DPH is accountable through a Director of Children's or Adult Services. This arrangement is viewed as unacceptable and as signalling a virtual demotion of the status of the public health function.

Perhaps the most significant change facing DsPH in the new structure is working in a political environment that is very different from the NHS one most previously inhabited. It has proved to be a source of considerable anxiety for many DsPH and it is acknowledged that they will need to be skilled at working in such an environment. In particular, this means working with and supporting local elected political leaders in their efforts to improve health. Indeed, working with elected members and influencing a wide range of partners both within the local authority and beyond will become the essence of a

DPH's remit. Some DsPH have already begun to operate in such a way, but, for others, the need to do so will present something of a challenge, especially those who have come from a clinical background and whose experience is largely confined to working within an NHS setting. These issues touch on some of the findings from our research, which pointed to the lack of understanding of different cultures despite a commitment to partnership working. In order to influence the agendas of a range of partners, an essential prerequisite is to understand their cultures and ways of behaving and doing business. Yet it remains the case that in general too little attention is given to this matter.

In order to discharge their responsibilities with minimal risk of their resources being raided or put to other uses, DsPH will preside over a ring-fenced public health budget. It is not certain how long such an arrangement will continue beyond 2015, if at all, but it will exist for at least a couple of years. Allocations to local authorities for the first two years of the new system, 2013/14 and 2014/15, were announced in January 2013, and although these have resulted in some poorer areas receiving less than they might merit and better-off areas receiving more, overall the settlement has resulted in higher allocations for all local authorities than was envisaged under the new formula and has been generally welcomed.

Views are decidedly mixed on the merits or otherwise of a ring-fenced budget for public health. There are those, principally existing DsPH and other practitioners, who fear that without guaranteed funding accompanying their move to local government, there can be no certainty that they will continue to have the wherewithal to maintain the essential public health services that local authorities will have a mandate to provide. But critics allege that DsPH will not make themselves popular by having a protected budget that is denied other local services, especially at a time of deep cuts in local government services, and that it will probably make relationship-building a tougher task than it might otherwise be.

It is hoped that DsPH will use their budgets, which will in any case be quite limited and tied to functions transferred to local government from the NHS, as leverage on other local authority services, with a view to increasing the overall investment in public health across councils. After all, it is argued, virtually all local government functions and services impact on public health in one way or another. It therefore makes sense to view all that a local authority does as having a public health dimension. This has led some local government leads, and other commentators, to propose a move to place-based or community budgets as soon as possible. These were experimented with in 2009/10 under the previous government in the form of an initiative known as Total Place Pilots. We return to this topic later.

Another concern in returning public health to local government is how far in fact meeting the 21st-century public health challenges entails action at a local level when most of the pressures on public health are in fact global and far beyond the reach of even nation states, never mind local authorities. This is especially the case in respect of tackling big corporate food and drink companies, whose actions may be said to determine lifestyle behaviour and the growing problem of obesity and alcohol misuse (Hastings, 2012). It may have been that in the Victorian era, it was possible for socially aware and committed individual medical practitioners, like John Snow and William Duncan, to make a significant and seminal impact on improving health, whether in the sphere of water quality and sewage disposal or the condition of housing. But, as we have seen from our earlier discussion, contemporary public health solutions are complex and demand attention at multiple levels, from the individual to transnational forums. This point was eloquently and painstakingly described in the 2007 Government Office for Science's Foresight report on obesity (Butland et al, 2007).

Of course, there is an important role for local government in reshaping what has been termed an obesogenic environment but it cannot achieve success in tackling obesity through its own efforts alone, with other measures required at higher levels of government. So, in moving public health back to local government, there is a question to be asked about how far public health issues can be tackled effectively at that level without appropriate action also occurring at other levels. Acknowledging that it cannot be left to localism to resolve these issues, Lang and Rayner (2012) call upon public health leaders working locally to 'be noisy and to build alliances'. Above all, they need to be 'change agents, building and supporting movements with agencies above and beyond the local' (Lang and Rayner, 2012).

It will fall to PHE, set up independently of the Department of Health as an arm's length executive agency, to provide national leadership for public health. PHE is responsible for health protection, emergency preparedness and the provision of public health information and evidence across all three domains of the public health function. On the latter function, it will work with the National Institute for Health and Clinical Excellence (NICE), rebranded the National Institute for Health and Care Excellence in April 2013 as a result of acquiring social care to add to its portfolio, and reconstituted as a non-departmental public body to confirm its independence from government. A considerable part of PHE's function involves working closely with local government, although quite how remains to be worked through. It will be important, as one witness giving evidence to the House of Commons Communities and Local Government Committee's inquiry into local authorities and health issues argued, for PHE to become more of an ally and 'critical friend' to local government rather than a regulator (Hughes, 2013). The operating model for PHE stresses that it will 'support local authorities in their new role by providing services, expertise, information and advice in a way that is responsive to local needs' (Department of Health, 2011b, p 2). It is accepted that PHE will not duplicate the work that local authorities do, but will focus its efforts on carrying out functions and activities that would not be practicable to replicate in every local authority. However, the test of all these fine words and reassurances will be how the relationship evolves in practice between local authorities, which have been around a long time, and PHE, which is the 'new kid on the block'.

PHE's independence has been an issue since under the initial proposals, it was to remain an agency located within the Department of Health. For the House of Commons Health Committee, in its inquiry into the new arrangements affecting public health, this was a major concern. It recommended that PHE 'must be – and, just as importantly, must be perceived as being – independent of the government. Only in this way will it maintain the reputation for independence and evidence-based expertise' (House of Commons Health Committee, 2011, p 23, para 61). The Committee believed that PHE must demonstrate that it is able to, and regularly does, speak 'truth unto power'.

Nationally, PHE comprises eight directorates and while most, if not all, of them will have some dealings with local authorities, three in particular are likely to have most contact: health protection; health improvement and population health; and knowledge and intelligence (Department of Health, 2012b).

Structurally, like NHS England, PHE has a regional and local presence (15 centres that deliver its locally facing services and act in support of local authorities). The four regions are coterminous with those for NHS England and the Department for Communities and Local Government's resilience hubs.

Apart from the central–local vertical relationship, there is also the national–national horizontal one to be sorted out. Given the split in responsibilities for aspects of public health between PHE and NHS England, especially affecting children and early years issues, there is a risk that their respective activities will not be as aligned as they ought to be. Unless this alignment occurs, then the problems we described in respect of our own research in regard to the impact of national policy on local partnerships and a failure to join it up could remain a problem. In particular, with responsibilities divided across the two national bodies and locally, the risk is that no one is in overall charge.

A second national–national horizontal relationship concerns the two central government departments that will preside over public health in varying degrees: the Department of Health, presumably in a somewhat truncated or diminished form given the creation of PHE; and the Department of Communities and Local Government, which oversees local government. These two departments have very different cultures and levels of understanding when it comes to both local government and public health. Little has been said about their relationship and yet it will be another critical factor in the mix if appropriately aligned national policy and consistent messages are to be communicated to local government. We know from the history of joined-up government, briefly reviewed in Chapter Two, that it has proved difficult to achieve in practice (Exworthy and Hunter, 2011).

Finally, removing the lead role for public health from the NHS to local government should not indicate or imply that the NHS no longer has a public health role. Given that the pressures on health services come largely from preventable lifestyle diseases, the NHS cannot ignore its responsibilities in making a difference through, for instance, the 'making every contact count' policy (NHS Future Forum, 2012). The question is how this is to be done if public health resources no longer exist in the NHS. The statutory offer of public health support to CCGs is obviously a key mechanism to ensure that the NHS retains a public health presence but if public health specialists continue to see their work focused on clinical commissioning priorities and evidence-based interventions as an integral part of their professional activity, then, as a witness to the Communities and Local Government Committee's inquiry put it: 'the fear is that this will quickly become a distraction from work on the wider determinants of health and lifestyle issues – the Marmot agenda' (Hughes, 2013). The risk is further compounded by the continued dominance of a medical model of health rather than a social model, which, for many, is the opportunity and grand prize offered by moving public health back to local government (Elson, 1999, 2004).

How the new arrangements will work in practice across the country is a major question to which there can be no definitive answer at this time. What is clear is that the new structures that have emerged are certainly no simpler than those that they have replaced, and are possibly more complex. Although local government has a lead role locally for public health, the two new national bodies, NHS England and PHE, will also have significant public health responsibilities. Working together both vertically and horizontally at a time when both bodies are still inventing themselves, and getting their respective structures and practices embedded, will be a huge challenge, especially with the commissioning function split between them and local government in the following ways:

- Local authorities will commission or provide public health and social care services, including: those for children aged between 5 and 19; health checks; some sexual health services; public mental health; physical activity; obesity; drug and alcohol misuse; and nutrition services. Links with the NHS for the delivery of some of these services will remain essential if fragmentation is to be avoided.

- PHE will be responsible for front-line health protection through its local centres. It will: commission or provide national prevention and early presentation campaigns; provide infectious disease prevention services and coordinate outbreak management programmes; deliver the emergency preparedness for and responses to flu pandemics; and provide health intelligence services, which were previously carried out by Public Health Observatories.

- NHS England will commission: public health services for children from pregnancy to age 5 (with responsibility for this due to transfer to local authorities in 2015); immunisation programmes; national screening programmes; public health care for people in prison and other places of detention; and sexual assault referral services.

When set out like this, it places the local government public health role in perspective, as does the disbursement of the £5 billion funding for public health, only £2 billion of which will go to local authorities – the rest being split between NHS England and PHE. Furthermore, of the sum going to local authorities, most of it has been identified as necessary spend for sexual health and substance misuse services, which are demand-led. It presents a problem for local authorities in terms of sufficient funds not being available to invest in prevention in areas like obesity and smoking cessation.

Obviously, some system to assess progress is required and the Department of Health published its public health outcomes framework in January 2012 (Department of Health, 2012c). This sets out the desired outcomes for public health and how these will be measured. There are two overarching outcomes: increased life expectancy, taking account of the quality as well as the length of life; and reduced differences in life expectancy and healthy life expectancy between communities through greater improvements in more disadvantaged communities. Outcomes are expected to be delivered through improvements across a broad range of public health indicators grouped into four domains relating to the three pillars of public health (health protection, health improvement and health care/public health):

- health protection;
- health improvement;
- healthcare/public health and preventing premature mortality; and
- improving the wider determinants of health.

The public health outcomes framework is to be used as a tool for local transparency and accountability, providing a means for benchmarking local progress within each local authority and across authorities, with a view to driving sector-led improvement (Department of Health and the Department for Communities and Local Government, 2013). Quite what the impact of the framework will be locally and how it will be used to monitor progress, identify gaps and provide an incentive to improve remains unclear in the absence of any single stakeholder assuming overall responsibility for its progress. After all, while local authorities may have been accorded the lead role for public health locally, the overall responsibility is split between local government, NHS England and PHE.

In setting out the new public health outcomes framework, the Department of Health is decidedly vague about where responsibility will lie for holding any of the partners to account for making progress (or not) in respect of the desired outcomes (Department of Health, 2012c). It simply states: 'Public Health England will support the Secretary of State in considering how the government can best achieve its strategic objectives across the system, working in partnership with local government and the NHS' (Department of Health, 2012c, p 7, para 1.7). However, what this will entail in practice remains unclear – as always, the devil is in the detail. Some clues, though, are given in the description of the outcomes framework. For example, it will be for local authorities, in partnership with HWBs, to demonstrate improvements in public health outcomes. It is envisaged that specific progress against the measures in the framework will be built into the joint strategic needs assessments (JSNAs) and joint health and wellbeing strategies (JHWSs), as appropriate.

PHE will have an important role in supporting the improvement of outcomes. It will have a primary role in delivering a number of the outcomes while also supporting local government in the achievement of others. In respect of the latter, PHE will publish tools that support benchmarking of outcomes between and within local areas to provide insights into performance. These may well have a number of common features, which resemble the Comprehensive Area Assessment (CAA) introduced by the Audit Commission and other regulatory bodies in 2009 but abolished after its first year of operation by the incoming Coalition government along with the Commission itself (Audit Commission et al, 2009).

The issue of sector-led improvement is a vexed one since local government cannot be performance-managed by central government although still needs to be held to account for its performance. Local authorities as elected bodies are ultimately accountable to their local communities. They are also free to set their priorities in accordance with local needs and preferences. But for central government, in the shape of the Department of Health and PHE, there will be anxieties concerning the degree to which health improvement occurs and health inequalities are tackled across the country in ways which do not widen the health gap or create what may become an unacceptable level of variation between different geographical areas, some of which already show marked differences. Local authorities, in seeking to improve their performance, tend to benchmark themselves against comparable local authorities. In addition, as the government noted in its response to the House of Commons Communities and Local Government Committee's report on the role of local authorities in health issues (Department of Health, 2013a), PHE will publish annual data in respect of each local authority against each of the indicators in the Public Health Outcomes Framework. PHE has also launched a website (Longer Lives) showing variations in death rates, which has met with a mixed response by some local authorities that worry about the value and impact of what they term 'league tables'. The website comes on the back of the Department of Health's call to action to reduce avoidable premature mortality (Department of Health, 2013b). This initiative is designed to provide local authorities and the NHS with an insight into the top causes of avoidable early deaths in their area and how they compare to other areas with a similar social and economic profile.

The issue of sector-led improvement is therefore a highly sensitive and delicate one, since there is wariness among local authorities over the purpose of such so-called 'league tables' and their intent. If it is to 'name and shame' local authorities that do not seem to be performing as well as their peers then there would be concern that such comparisons were being made without a full appreciation of the context and circumstances that might be contributing to such an outcome. Also, at a time when new relationships are being formed between PHE and local authorities, it will be of critical importance to ensure that these are built on trust if they are to be mutually productive. It is Hughes' point noted earlier about PHE being seen to be a 'critical friend' rather than a regulator (Hughes, 2013).

New public health partnerships

As mentioned, the arrangements for public health introduced in April 2013 have required new partnerships to be introduced, which, in most cases, will replace those that have existed hitherto. However, Local Strategic Partnerships (LSPs) are likely to continue in some places, which could cause confusion since they are not dissimilar bodies to the new principal partnership mechanism, HWBs, in terms of their membership, remit and focus on integration and joint working. Overlapping membership between LSPs and HWBs could also cause unnecessary duplication. However, in the main, the establishment of HWBs has meant new structures and personnel and while these changes can in some respects be seen as energising and reinvigorating the whole notion of partnership working, what it means and how it can be strengthened by learning the lessons from past failed partnerships, they also pose significant issues at an especially challenging time for those charged with the task of making the changes work. Certainly, most of those giving evidence to the House of Commons Communities and Local Government Committee's inquiry into the role of local authorities in health issues expressed optimism that the new arrangements held considerable promise, with a few witnesses urging caution against expecting too much of them too soon (House of Commons Communities and Local Government Committee, 2013).

HWBs, for the most part, replace previous arrangements designed to enable the NHS and local government to improve public health through the coordination of the NHS, social care and public health at a local level. Under the Health and Social Care Act 2012, upper-tier local authorities and unitary authorities have a statutory duty to create an HWB and develop a new JHWS, which will be informed by a JSNA. Between them, JSNAs and JHWSs will form the basis of the NHS's and local authorities' own commissioning plans across health and social care, public health, and some children's services. As we reported from our research, JSNAs were not regarded as terribly effective in driving the partnership agenda or local priorities prior to the current changes. The Department of Health and Department for Communities and Local Government, in their joint submission to the House of Commons Communities and Local Government Committee's inquiry, describe HWBs as being 'the forum for local authorities, the NHS, local Healthwatch, communities and wider partners, to share system leadership of both health and care services and population health' (Department of Health and Department for Communities and Local Government, 2013).

HWBs are possibly the one change that has met with overwhelming support from various quarters, although whether this optimism is justified or not remains largely untested. They seem to have the 'X factor' in terms of their popularity and high hopes that they can achieve great things. Expectations are running high, possibly absurdly so, which will not help HWBs find their place. An early implementers programme was launched by the Department of Health in 2011, which led to most local areas setting up HWBs. These operated in shadow form across the country for some time prior to their formal commencement in April 2013. There is no standard model as, in keeping with the spirit of localism, the HWBs have been encouraged to establish their own membership and devise a working arrangement that is best suited to their particular local circumstances. While local areas have been enthusiastic about establishing HWBs, there are as many types as there are HWBs. They come in all shapes and sizes and have very different conceptions of what their purpose is and how they intend to achieve it. Letting a thousand flowers bloom has been encouraged, with the Department of Health resisting calls to prescribe a model for HWBs. However, the Act does prescribe a minimum membership requirement of at least one councillor, the director of adult social services, the director of children's services, the director of public health, a representative of the local Healthwatch organisation – another new body introduced to strengthen public involvement – a representative of each relevant CCG, and such others as the local authority thinks appropriate. NHS England must also participate in HWBs when invited to do so. Separately, the national director for the implementation of HWBs recommended a membership size of between eight and 10 members to ensure that the HWBs are 'change agents' (Department of Health, 2011a). A serious perceived lacuna in the membership of HWBs is the absence of district council members. In practice, many local authorities have put in place arrangements to engage district councils, which is entirely proper given that these councils provide vital services affecting public health, such as spatial planning, environmental health and recreation.

A great deal rests on HWBs. The House of Commons Communities and Local Government Committee concluded that they have a pivotal role and their success 'is crucial to the new arrangements'; but it also warned of the danger 'that the initial optimism surrounding their establishment and first year or two in operation will falter and go the way of previous attempts at partnership working that failed and became no more than expensive talking shops' (House of Commons Communities and Local Government Committee, 2013, p 14, para 22). Reaffirming key findings from our own research, the Committee maintained that success would be contingent on HWBs working 'on the basis of relationships and influence', which would depend on both people and structures. However, while this may be the right approach, it is likely to 'make demands on local authorities' leadership and relationship-building skills' (House of Commons Communities and Local Government Committee, 2013, p 14, para 22).

An interim assessment of progress

The public health changes are both extensive and complex and will take time to settle in as new relationships are formed. There are many new organisations and interfaces to be negotiated, all of which will take time and require well-developed boundary-spanning skills. At the centre of all the changes are HWBs. They come with great hopes attached to them but it will be some time before a reliable or convincing verdict can be offered on whether the new HWBs can rise to the many challenges confronting them and realise these hopes. In the meantime, informed commentary on their challenges is not in short supply and offers some illuminating insights into what might be expected over time.

In particular, reflecting at least in part an awareness of the great expectations of them, there is a desire among many HWBs to do partnership working differently and to avoid the bureaucratic impasse that many of their predecessors ended up in. Our research, reported in Chapters Four and Five, documented many of these problems and also provided some pointers for future partnership working. While it may be the case that some HWBs have heeded these lessons and attended to the evidence, it is much more likely that HWBs have pursued their own preferences and are at risk of repeating many of the mistakes previous partnerships have made, which sealed their fate. Certainly, an early assessment of HWBs warned about the danger of them becoming another 'talking shop' and of failing to ensure that their strategic vision was fulfilled (Humphries et al, 2012). That is the crux of the issue: will HWBs be the system leaders their supporters hope for, or will they become mere talking shops, which risk becoming marginalised as decisions get taken elsewhere? It has also been argued that HWBs that look and behave like traditional local authority committees will risk repeating the mistakes of previous partnership boards and fail as a result (Humphries, 2013). In short, for the new HWBs to succeed, they must be different.

In his written evidence to the House of Commons Communities and Local Government Committee's inquiry, a former DPH and head of the now-defunct National Support Team on Health Inequalities at the Department of Health was sceptical as to whether HWBs were up to the job (Bentley, 2013). The governance issue particularly vexed him since it was not clear who was running the show and who would be held to account, and by whom, for implementing the JHWS each HWB would be responsible for producing. The performance management dimension, as distinct from acting as a strategic forum, was unclear. Bentley believes that acting as a strategic forum adds little value if there is no mechanism for being clear about what has changed as a result of the HWB selecting a particular priority, or if organisations cannot be held to account by the HWB for their contribution, or if there is not a clear sense of how joint working has made change possible. He is critical of HWBs that plan to meet quarterly since that is unlikely to enable the necessary momentum to be generated and maintained. He asks: 'How can the large and complex agenda of health and wellbeing for any population be done justice? How can the HWB become the "beating heart" of local process for improving health and wellbeing?' (Bentley, 2013). If this concern is coupled with concerns about membership being large and agendas being long, then the future for HWBs does not look terribly inspiring or optimistic.

Although, in these evolving arrangements, Bentley is able to point to some examples where such issues are being acknowledged and addressed, overall he remains concerned that 'many local arrangements are not coming together with the definition and precision in governance necessary to generate step changes in population health and wellbeing' (Bentley, 2013). Part of the problem lies in poor JSNAs, which, despite being in existence for a few years, Bentley believes have remained 'patchy and variable', with a number of which merely being recycled for a new year under the new HWBs. He claims that few HWBs are managing to achieve the 'uneasy balancing act' that involves combining 'top-down, largely quantitative analysis with bottom-up more qualitative intelligence, concerns and opinions from communities and frontline staff' (Bentley, 2013). This is a particularly important point given the research we presented in Chapters Four and

Five demonstrating the absence of effective joining-up between the strategic and front-line levels in many partnerships.

In a report by the Smith Institute (Churchill, 2012), contributors agree that HWBs are central to the government's vision of a more integrated approach to health and social care. But therein lies a danger, for if HWBs become preoccupied by the health and social care conundrum that has defeated both the NHS and social care for the past 50 years or so, then their impact on public health will be lost. It is all too easy to foresee this danger occurring. The provision of social care occupies around 80% of local government spending and many local authorities predict that with severe cuts affecting their services, within a few years, local government may be providing little else but social care. Also, the NHS is under pressure (and not for the first time) to clear acute beds, about 70% of which are occupied by elderly people who have no need of them other than there is nowhere else for them to go. In comparison with the short-term pressures from this sector, compounded by a government committed to integrated care, the move to improve public health is unlikely to be regarded as so urgent or the top priority for cash-strapped local authorities and other public services. Indeed, one witness giving evidence to the House of Commons Communities and Local Government inquiry considered that 'the construction of HWBs is largely to do with the NHS and adult social care interface' (House of Commons Communities and Local Government Committee, 2013, p 16, para 26). Scally went on to express his fear 'that public health concerns and the overall health of the population will lose out' (House of Commons Communities and Local Government Committee, 2013, p 16, para 26).

The risk of HWBs being hijacked by the health and social care agenda was noted by the House of Commons Communities and Local Government Committee. While acknowledging the 'substantial mandate to encourage integrated working between the NHS and public health', the Committee stresses the need 'to maintain a strategic and balanced outlook on their new responsibilities, focusing on promoting the health of their local population, rather than becoming exclusively preoccupied with the detail of health and social care commissioning and integration' (House of Commons Communities and Local Government Committee, 2013, p 16, para 26).

The risk facing HWBs has been heightened by the government's plans being consulted upon to 'refresh' its mandate to NHS England (Department of Health, 2013c). There is concern, expressed by its policy director, that in some areas the government's proposed changes move 'into the territory of "how" the NHS should deliver rather than focusing on the more strategic question of what outcomes it should achieve' (McCarthy, 2013). This creates the risk that the 'additional burden on the health system and focus on process measures will reduce the ability of its ... health and wellbeing partners to respond effectively to the health outcomes and inequalities that are most important locally'. Much of the refreshing of the mandate is concerned with removing the barriers to integration following the decision to invest £3.8 billion of NHS funding into pooled budgets to bring about deeper integration between health and social care. If the revised mandate goes ahead as proposed then it is likely there would be an impact on HWBs and where they might be under pressure to place their priorities.

Despite the considerable pressures on HWBs to do things differently, which carry the inevitable risk that they will fail, there remains optimism in many quarters that a new and innovative approach is taking root. For Rogers, Chair of the Community Wellbeing Board at the Local Government Association, HWBs are 'the single most important component of the new health landscape' (Rogers, 2012, p 28). However, if the new HWBs are to succeed, it will require a radical new approach, with partnership working moving from being regarded as a 'marginal activity to the main way of doing business' (Rogers, 2012, p 28). Echoing some of the lessons from our own research reported in Chapters Four and Five, Rogers believes that the only way to achieve success this time round:

> is by moving our focus from structures and processes to outcomes and relationship building. HWBs are the primary means through which we will agree on shared outcomes and build strong relationships.... It will take considerable skill for HWBs to hold the ring in this complex system of relationships. (Rogers, 2012, p 28)

For a start, HWBs will have on them as co-equals elected members and officers who will not have worked together previously in such a way. Hitherto, officers have been advisers to elected members. Some of the HWBs are chaired by elected members (often the council's health lead) and they face new challenges in respect of how they balance the politics of place, their democratic mandate and their new responsibility for the collective leadership of the HWB. Rogers fears that faced with such complex issues, many HWBs might be tempted to retreat into their comfort zone 'by focusing on structures, governance and constitutional architecture for the board' (Rogers, 2012, p 30), which was the default position favoured by many of their predecessors.

To avoid such an outcome, many HWBs, actively supported by the Local Government Association and others, are investing in leadership and organisation development. However, it remains a risk, especially as some HWB members have only recently joined, since getting the two national bodies, NHS England and PHE, established and up and running has taken much longer than envisaged, with the result that many posts in the new structures have only recently been filled. This is especially the case in respect of PHE, which only completed making its senior national staff appointments at the end of 2012 and has spent most of 2013 putting in place the new sub-national structures and systems.

Locally, HWBs will need to work closely with CCGs, especially if the JHWSs to be produced by the HWBs are not to run foul of CCG commissioning preferences and decisions. Though unlikely, if CCGs should choose to reject a JHWS, then it can be referred to NHS England, but this will incur lengthy delays and is probably an outcome to be avoided if at all possible. There is also a risk of HWBs getting too close to CCGs or, as the Royal Town Planning Institutes warns in written evidence to the Communities and Local Government Committee, being seen as a secondary body to CCGs and thereby neglecting their key role 'in shaping the wider determinants of health, and in promoting other services that impact on public health (e.g. land use planning, green space and transport)' (Royal Town Planning Institute, 2013).

Issues concerning HWBs were a central topic of interest in the House of Commons Communities and Local Government Committee's inquiry into the role of local authorities in health (House of Commons Communities and Local Government Committee, 2013). Both the written and oral evidence submitted to the Committee testified to a number of concerns over HWBs and the high expectations of them, which, as noted earlier, could prove to be unrealistic. One council leader expressed a worry that, while welcoming HWBs, their very existence could result in other ways of intervening to improve health and wellbeing being overlooked. Local authority engagement in spatial planning, regulation and supporting communities to mobilise their own assets should not suffer with the arrival of HWBs.

But another witness giving oral evidence spoke of local government not always having the confidence to use the many levers available to it for improving health, including education, housing and transport (Hicks, 2013). He hoped that with public health having returned to local government, it would raise its game and 'put the improvement of the health of their population and the narrowing of health inequalities right at the core of their purpose' (Hicks, 2013). For another witness, while supporting the return of public health to local government, he did not consider it to be a 'full return' (Scally, 2013b). When the allocation of responsibilities was studied, a substantial number lay at national level with NHS England and PHE.

Another witness, Independent Chair of Oldham's Shadow HWB, reinforced the big risk raised earlier that 'issues related to health and social care provision will "crowd out" attention to the wider determinants of health and the urgent need for changes in lifestyle and behaviour' (Hughes, 2013). This is a worry that permeates much of the written and oral evidence received by the Committee. The UK Healthy Cities Network, for example, made the point 'that HWBs should be about governance *for* health, not just the governance *of* health (services)' (UK Healthy Cities Network, 2013). Also, the former Regional Director of Public Health for NHS South West, Gabriel Scally, wrote in his written evidence that the remit of HWBs consulted upon by the Department of Health 'is very disappointing in that it concentrates on the commissioning of services'. He believes that 'this will have the effect of concentrating attention on the social care–NHS interface and lead to the relative neglect of health improvement and the importance of action on the wider determinants of health' (Scally, 2013a).

But it is not just the NHS–social care interface that could preoccupy HWBs or absorb the bulk of their time and effort. With the NHS having radically to transform services to save funds for reinvestment elsewhere, major issues loom on the horizon in regard to hospital reconfiguration and mergers. Traditionally, such issues go to the heart of local community concerns about the future of the NHS. Highly charged local campaigns are the usual response, with all the political and emotional heat that goes with them. It is inconceivable that HWBs, unless they are exceptionally focused and disciplined, will be able to avoid being sucked into such issues even if they wanted to. Indeed, under the existing permissive arrangements, some HWBs are unclear about their role in relation to acute sector provision, while others see a very clear role for themselves in influencing hospital commissioning. The risk is one of further 'crowding out' of the wider public health agenda.

The Royal Town Planning Institute, in its written evidence to the Communities and Local Government Committee, believes that health services:

> can act as a springboard for wider economic regeneration of an area. Encouraging health services to relocate to town and district centres within communities is a positive step as

these areas are in most cases already served by good transport links. (Royal Town Planning Institute, 2013)

But for such an approach to succeed, local authorities and their HWBs will need to view health care services needs as shaping outcomes beyond those that are seen to be traditional improvements in health.

Hughes, in his written evidence to the Communities and Local Government Committee, also echoed the findings from our research on partnerships when he observed that despite several positive examples of bringing people together to generate health improvement across complex systems, 'the evidence about partnership working has often been disappointing. There is limited evidence about partnerships producing sustained health improvement, nor have they been able to move much investment upstream' (Hughes, 2013). He therefore concludes, somewhat pessimistically, that it is 'an act of faith that HWBs will be able to generate better outcomes for population health and service integration' (Hughes, 2013). For him, a key success indicator of HWBs will be the scale of redirecting investment upstream into prevention.

Adopting a whole system partnership approach was regarded by another witness as essential. In his written evidence he asserted that 'the aim of such an approach 'is to secure shared understanding, priorities and alignment of national and local agendas underpinned by shared values and the collective use of resources to deliver' (Grady, 2013). The leadership role of local government should take the form of being an orchestrator of these new partnerships. Reinforcing a point made by others, Grady claimed that 'the aim must be a new direction for local authorities ... with a focus on partnership working' (Grady, 2013). He made reference to the Total Place initiative introduced under the Labour government in 2009/10, with the aim of removing contradictions between different policies and reducing inefficiencies and duplication between programmes (HM Treasury and Department of Communities and Local Government, 2010). The initiative involved a number of pilots across England and while it did not have sufficient time to prove itself, early indications were that the approach was showing promising improvements for local populations (Humphries and Gregory, 2010; Grint, 2010). This suggests that the continued focus on place-based service planning and delivery through community budgets offers an opportunity to use resources more flexibly across services.

There are other potential pitfalls facing HWBs and the principal ones have been highlighted by Humphries et al (2012) in their early review of the HWBs in shadow form. Despite the rhetoric of localism, which is allegedly the whole point of the changes and the new Act, many HWBs in their shadow form expressed concern that national policy imperatives would override locally agreed priorities and they were uncertain about the extent to which they would be able to influence decisions of NHS England. A similar issue may arise over PHE once it gets fully into gear. For local authorities not used to an NHS command-and-control management culture, this will come as something of a shock, though not one that they are likely to put up with for long should it become a problem. Roles and responsibilities in respect of all the new bodies will need to be more clearly defined than is so far apparent. However, the point bears out one of the key findings from our research, namely, that local partnerships are not immune from national policy concerns and how these get played out in terms of the expectations placed on local agencies when it comes to implementation.

The issue of policy alignment, convergence and coherence, and the need for it at the various levels of government, is critical. As we noted earlier in this chapter, it is an issue elsewhere in Europe, too, as the WHO report on local government's role in improving health showed (Grady and Goldblatt, 2012). Without such alignment, learning from success and spreading and sharing it become much more difficult to achieve. The risk is that scaling up local initiatives into national objectives fails to occur and small-scale initiatives slip back to focusing on lifestyles and behaviour change, leaving the social determinants, which may be beyond any single local authority to address on its own, pretty much intact. Part of the leadership challenge is ensuring that there is policy synergy and coherence not only horizontally at the various levels, but also vertically between them. In the context of the new changes to public health being implemented in England, it will be a particular challenge given the raft of existing and new bodies now in place.

The organisational architecture is certainly more complicated than the arrangements they have replaced. Whereas nationally, there were two central departments overseeing the NHS and local government, respectively, albeit operating within very different cultures and contexts, since April 2013, these two bodies have been joined by two new ones, NHS England and PHE, which will enjoy considerably more independence, especially the former. Ensuring effective join-up between all four organisations is going to be a huge challenge and, it has to be said, the lessons from previous efforts at joined-up government do not inspire much confidence that things will be so different in future (Hunter, 2003; Parker et al, 2010; Exworthy and Hunter, 2011). As the Institute for Government's critique of the fragmented nature of Whitehall suggests, if there has been negligible progress in achieving more effective joined-up working locally, then much of the blame lies in the centre's inability to be joined up: 'So long as departmentalism at the centre remains a problem [m]ore effective local coordination' is no substitute (Parker et al, 2010, p 93). In particular, as the Institute and others have concluded, 'wicked' issues, such as alcohol misuse and childhood obesity, have defied successive attempts at making joined-up government a reality. In the absence of stronger incentives to collaborate, along the lines perhaps of place-based budgeting, it is hard to see how or why things should change. However, for initiatives like Total Place to succeed requires central government to let go and adopt some of the joined-up thinking that is happening locally (Exworthy and Hunter, 2011).

Besides having to manage the possibility of policy misalignment and incoherence and a lack of convergence, other risks to HWBs arise from their very diversity and newness since different approaches and models will emerge, some of which will almost certainly be more successful than others. It will be important to capture and share learning and also to allow for failure. The problem is that it will take time for HWBs to succeed, and time is not on the side of impatient policymakers anxious for signs of quick results, especially in the run-up to the next election in 2015. The NHS and, to a lesser extent, public health changes have, as we pointed out earlier, not been at all popular and the fact that the government went ahead in the face of widespread opposition to force them through Parliament remains a source of deep and continuing anger and resentment. Having virtually expended its political capital, the government desperately needs to be able to point to some good news to justify the turmoil it has put services and staff through. Given that it acknowledges that the return of public health to local government was one of its least unpopular proposals, it will be eagerly anticipating some quick pay-off. However, the changes are occurring in a wider environment that is less than auspicious; hence the suggestion that they may amount to a poisoned chalice for local government rather than the new dawn many had hoped. Unprecedented financial pressures, rising demand from an ageing and to some extent unhealthier population across the age range but especially among young people, and complex organisational changes affecting all public services could amount to a perfect storm. At the very least, the convergence of these pressures will severely test local authorities' political leadership.

A further test of the new arrangements will arise in regard to how far local authorities are able to take a strategic look across their responsibilities. The point is prompted by a King's Fund study showing that, to date, the government has sought to tackle unhealthy behaviours in silos, that is, producing separate strategies for obesity, smoking and alcohol that do not link to each other or to policies on health inequalities (Buck and Frosini, 2012). The study also shows – although it is not an especially novel finding since the argument has been made before and known for some time – that unhealthy behaviours co-occur and cluster in population groups, particularly those most disadvantaged. Truly joined-up policy would acknowledge such connections across public health issues and those most affected by them. It is the way professions are trained and organised and government departments function largely in separate silos that encourages a silo-based approach, which ignores the evidence suggesting a more effective approach might be to tackle the causes rather than the symptoms. The King's Fund study found that, in 2003, people with the lowest levels of formal education were three times more likely not to adhere to government guidelines on all four chief unhealthy behaviours (ie smoking, alcohol, diet, physical activity). By 2008, they were five times more likely not to adhere to the guidelines. It is little wonder that policy has failed and inequalities in health have widened (National Audit Office, 2010b).

The final question, and possibly most important of all, is whether HWBs will have sufficient powers and authority to make a difference. Conceivably, their significant responsibilities and the high expectations placed on them are not matched by the powers accorded them. The Royal College of Nursing, in its evidence to the Communities and Local Government Committee makes the perfectly valid point that while the statutory existence of HWBs is an important advance, their strategic role and powers 'are, in truth, similar to those of previous arrangements' (Royal College of Nursing, 2013). The Royal College of Nursing is especially concerned that the powers and influence of HWBs in relation to CCGs 'may not be sufficiently robust in legislation. It remains to be seen whether HWBs will have any real power in challenging commissioning decisions, or how or what action [NHS England] will take in local disputes' (Royal College of Nursing, 2013).

Conclusion

At the time of writing, it is not possible to pass judgement on the changes that have been introduced either to public health generally or to public health partnerships in particular. The jury remains firmly out. Once again, public health finds itself at a critical juncture. There is certainly the potential for the new arrangements to deliver progress of a kind and on a scale that has been eluded public health for the most part when the function was located within the NHS family. With few exceptions, it remained in the shadows of a largely clinically dominated, hospital-focused service – as the late Derek Wanless commented in his report on public health for the government in 2004 (Wanless, 2004) and others have analysed (Hunter, 2003).

But while local government should in theory offer a more sympathetic, supportive and generally more appropriate and logical setting to improve health through approaches that were difficult to justify or get supported in an NHS context, there remain significant barriers to progress. Some of these involve revisiting, and taking heed of, the lessons from our own research and whether these have been learned or are likely to be. We return to these in Chapter Seven. However, others arise from the overall political, economic and social context, which has changed considerably in the past few years, especially in England. The place of public services in society, how they are to be provided in future, if at all, and by whom are fundamental questions that were not even being asked when our research on partnerships was being carried out. Similarly, the move to end the public provision of services and replace them with private sector alternatives, and chiefly of a for-profit nature, is another development that has gone much further in the past couple of years or so than was envisaged or foreseen (Gash et al, 2013). Whatever the future shape of the landscape, and the types of architecture that are erected upon it to carry out the public health function, partnership working will be required, but whether HWBs are the optimum mechanism for the task, only time will tell. There is certainly hope and optimism that they might be, but also fears that expectations of them may be running unrealistically and unreasonably high. As one commentator put it, 'cynics would not be surprised if their remit is extended to achieving world peace on the grounds that this is a slightly less challenging task than the remit in their own backyard' (Humphries, 2013).

SEVEN

Conclusion: the future for public health partnerships

Partnerships have never been out of vogue in UK public policy – and certainly not in recent times – but the need for them has arguably never been greater. This poses something of a paradox, with which our study has been concerned. The silo-based departmental culture and character of the UK, but especially English, system of government at both national and local levels has triggered a continuing interest in partnerships to overcome the worst effects of working in silos. However, few partnerships have succeeded altogether in overcoming the silo effect or departmentalism mindset. For the most part, partnerships represent another layer of governance, or 'add-on', and a patchy and uneven one at that in terms of their effectiveness, as the findings from our study of public health partnerships show. On the few occasions where partnerships appear to work well, there are many more instances where the costs may outweigh the benefits – at least those that can be ascribed to the partnership arrangements in place, which is not an easy calculation to make.

Given the enormity of the fiscal challenges facing all parts of the public sector over the coming years, the strengths and weaknesses of the new arrangements put in place from April 2013, following the passage of the Health and Social Care Act a year earlier in March 2012, will be tested to the limit. It is, of course, far too soon to offer a verdict on, or even to predict, the likely success of these new partnerships, which principally revolve around Health and Wellbeing Boards (HWBs), but it is a fair bet that unless they do operate in a quite different fashion from those that have preceded them, then in seeking to tackle the cross-cutting 'wicked issues' of the type to be found in public health, for the most part, they will be found wanting. But there does now exist a sizeable body of literature and learning upon which to draw that offers the new HWBs a real opportunity to avoid the path dependency option and to strike out in a new direction. Certainly, the overwhelming weight of oral and written evidence submitted to the House of Commons Communities and Local Government Committee's inquiry into the role of local authorities in health issues both acknowledged the opportunities facing HWBs and drew attention to the lessons from past attempts at partnership working. If nothing else, there is evidence of a more sophisticated discourse around partnerships and an acceptance that success hinges upon more than getting the structures and governance arrangements right, important though these may be. However, they are not sufficient in themselves.

Research findings, including those from our own study, point to the need for much greater clarity and rigour in the way partnerships are formed, led and performance-managed, although given the complex nature of public health problems, this is unlikely to be straightforward or even always possible. The systems perspective we have adopted in our own work suggests the need for a rather different approach in regard to how partnership working is conceived and pursued. We have drawn on the literature that describes wicked issues as being characterised by poor 'focus' and limited agreement about what exactly the problems are, and by uncertainty and ambiguity about how they might best be tackled. Wicked issues are invariably complex and rather messy, sitting outside single departments or silos and often sprawling across systems. They are not tame and neither are they merely complicated. Yet, they are precisely the sort of problems that partnerships are set up to confront. Our research suggests that such complex, dynamic and interdependent 'tangles', as they have been called, have no correct or even lasting solutions (Edmonstone, 2010). In such a context, most of our current thinking about partnership working falls short of what is required to make effective inroads into a series of wicked issues, which are often interconnected, that is, the issue of obesity, say, may be embedded in the issue of health inequalities (Buck and Frosini, 2012), or, as we saw in one of our research study sites, the issue of teenage pregnancy may be inextricably linked to alcohol misuse. However, instead of adopting a continually reflexive and self-examining approach, managers are, or feel, compelled to establish structures and mechanisms based on tools and guidance that risks them becoming deskilled. Yet, what may actually be required are '"clumsy" solutions that avoid a search for perfection and seek to "craft" a way forward by pragmatic negotiation, bargaining and a system-wide approach embodying working in partnership with other groups and agencies' (Edmonstone, 2010, p 228). A similar argument is advanced by Abrahamson and Freedman (2006) in their critique of the bias towards neatness. Their case is that too much neatness can lead to 'over-organisation', which can be as much of a problem as too little. They suggest that there is:

> an optimal level of mess for every aspect of every system. That is, in any situation there is a type and level of mess

at which effectiveness is maximised, and our assertion is
that people and organisations frequently err on the side of
overorganisation. (Abrahamson and Freedman, 2006, p 53)

Mess, they make clear, has little to do with chaos theory or complexity
thinking, which do not subscribe to pure randomness, but rather seek
order in phenomena. In contrast, mess is simply a lack of order, but
it may be of significance to how people and organisations function.
Abrahamson and Freedman (2006, pp 78–9) identify six benefits that
messiness can confer: flexibility, completeness, resonance, invention,
efficiency and robustness. Of these, a major benefit is flexibility, which
is to be found in numerous situations. For example, jazz improvisation
enables a group of musicians to shift at any moment to address an
audience's response to the music, and an organisational chart that is not
overly rigid and does not lock employees down into tightly defined
specialities and job roles can make it easier to reconfigure resources
around new challenges.

However, it is hard, if not inconceivable, in our system of government
to operate in such a flexible manner; one that sees value in taking risks
through the adoption of a 'suck it and see' approach which might mean
that mistakes are made. Even when the Coalition government seeks
to devolve responsibility to allow, if not encourage, innovation and
diversity, as it is seeking to do via its focus on localism, the powerful
centrifugal forces reassert themselves before long and efforts to break
out of this straightjacket become mere rhetorical devices concealing
a reality that tells a rather different story. A casual observer only has to
scan the endless outpourings from central government departments and
their agencies in the form of guidance and advice to see that little has
substantively changed. While often presented as non-prescriptive and
designed to be helpful and developmental, there is a thin line between
what is regarded as permissive and what rapidly becomes the expected
response and way of behaving in regard to how that guidance or advice
is acted upon. We return to these issues later.

Although there was little hint of this in the run-up to the election,
the arrival in office of a new UK government (in May 2010) was
accompanied by constant references to the parlous state of the economy,
in particular, the significant current account deficit, as cover for major,
if not unprecedented, public sector reform, including the NHS and
local government. Reform of this nature, and on such a scale and in
a largely hostile political and economic environment, poses both risks
and opportunities when it comes to addressing many of the issues
raised by our research.

As we have seen in Chapter Six, some believe that the reforms bring a new opportunity to learn the lessons from past failed or poorly performing partnerships, in order to put in place fresh and innovative approaches that incremental reform would not have achieved. However, others assert that the upheaval can only result in the loss from public health of valuable networks, relationships and expertise, with the consequence that new partnerships will have to be formed all over again and the risk that old mistakes are merely repeated. Furthermore, the 'corporate memory' of organisations and a lot of trust and goodwill – the glue that holds partnerships together – will have been lost. This is in addition to the loss of progress and the amount of time it will take these new bodies to find their feet and start delivering tangible health outcomes.

We also highlighted that an early assessment of the newly created HWBs cautioned against the danger of them becoming talking shops and failing to fulfil their strategic vision (Humphries et al, 2012). It was noted that there is also a concern that HWBs risk becoming marginalised as decisions get taken elsewhere, since they are not executive bodies, but have power only to produce health and wellbeing strategies. While rejecting these might be risky, and for the most part unlikely, there remains a more general problem with strategies of this kind, which at least one seasoned senior public health practitioner has dismissed as being 'pink and fluffy' (House of Commons Communities and Local Government Committee, 2013, Ev 54). If strategies of this type are commonplace, then it will be easy in practice to quietly ignore them. However, as we also pointed out in Chapter Six, an even bigger risk facing HWBs is that they become hijacked by immediate NHS concerns over hospital closures and mergers or with integrated care issues centred on health and social care, which will push public health priorities to the outer edge of what needs to be done. With an election looming in 2015, a government fixated on integrated care and an NHS desperate to make savings, it does not take a lot of political savvy to know where the focus of attention is likely to lie. Therefore, the greater risk to HWBs is that they are not in fact public health partnerships at all, but partnerships of a much narrower type that are devoted to addressing issues at the interface between health and social care.

As our research shows, many of the issues that have exercised partnership working in general over the years appear to apply and remain alive in the context of public health partnerships. This is the case both now and in the future, as changes in the NHS and local government are implemented. Despite the introduction of various new structures and systems, these appear to be of secondary importance in determining whether or not partnerships are perceived to be effective. Of greater importance is the existence (or absence) of trust and of relational issues among those engaged in partnerships and trying to make them work. If these are strong and well developed, then the perception, at least, is that partnerships work better and stand a chance of making real progress. The word 'goodwill' was mentioned several times by many participants in our study and was a key element of the systematic literature review conducted as part of the research. Some of those in our sample of study sites provided examples of where this had occurred. However, it seemed a rather fragile basis on which to build and sustain partnerships, especially when they were subject to constant policy and organisational churn and buffeting.

Another key theme from the research is that whatever the weaknesses and limitations of partnerships, they are perceived to be essential if public health issues are to be tackled. We were repeatedly told that the complex and multifaceted nature of such issues makes it inconceivable and impractical for any single agency to assume sole responsibility for making progress. Few of our interviewees offered any suggestions or proposals for new ways of tackling either partnerships or the issues with which they were grappling. Yet, from what we were told by many of those working at the front line, it does seem as if a loosening up of partnerships locally to allow and encourage different approaches may be worth considering. However, as we highlighted earlier, there is a danger of HWBs proceeding in the same path-dependent fashion and the same mistakes, notably, an emphasis on structures and processes, being replicated.

Looking to the future

Looking to the future, and in particular at the government's plans for changes in the public health function, it seems certain that partnership working is going to become even more complex and challenging. Two reasons for this merit particular comment and were mentioned by many of those who took part in our research. First, with an increasing diversity of service providers being encouraged, and with public health interventions involving private (for-profit and not-for-profit) companies becoming more active, the composition and nature of partnerships is likely to change and come to resemble public–private rather than public–public partnerships. Examples of these are already evident in the spheres of procurement and capital-building projects and in aspects of social care. They remain the exception in regard to public health but the situation is almost certain to change, with implications for the issues considered in this research. A particular concern expressed by some of our interviewees related to the tensions evident in working collaboratively in an increasingly competitive environment. Resolving, or perhaps at best managing, these tensions is likely to be one of the major challenges confronting partnerships in future.

Second, as part of the mixed economy of health that is being actively encouraged in England, the role of the voluntary, or third, sector is expected to grow, with new organisational forms in respect of cooperatives and social enterprises developing rapidly. There is a long tradition of voluntary sector engagement in partnership working but the expectations of this sector, and the heavy demands being placed on it in the planning and delivery of services, have grown enormously in the past few years. This, as many of our research respondents told us, is putting a considerable strain on their slender resources and leadership capacity. All this is also in addition to the cuts taking their toll on the third sector as part of the government's austerity measures (Wilding, 2010). Ironically, for a government ostensibly committed to local groups and communities taking over and running previously publicly run services, its policies seem deliberately designed to hamper and obstruct such activity rather than encourage and facilitate it. As a result, many third sector bodies are at risk, both financially and because they are unable to compete for service contracts with their much larger and smarter for-profit counterparts.

However, although partnership working may become more complex and challenging in future, its design may also become more local and context-specific, which, from our research, is a development we consider has many strengths, although this should not be at the expense of central government acknowledging its responsibilities for tackling public health issues at a level that only governments can do. From the findings to emerge from our research, especially those coming from service users and many front-line practitioners, there might be merit in trying to simplify structures and processes so that they are more joined-up and have a clearer focus on achievable outcomes, however modest. This may, in turn, enable partnerships to become more flexible and responsive to public health challenges, which would seem desirable given the constantly changing nature of these in the light of new policies and structures, and also the emergence of new knowledge and evidence about what may be effective.

Such an alternative approach might be based on themed or issue-based partnerships involving only those stakeholders directly involved with the particular public health issue, or theme, being addressed. They would be tasked with tackling a specific objective and would replace the catch-all, and potentially cumbersome, partnership body made up of all interested parties in an effort to be inclusive. Themed partnerships would need to be clear about their goals and how they would be delivered, by whom and by when. They might also need to be time-limited in order to avoid them becoming entrenched and fossilised. They would need to include, and also release, stakeholders as and when appropriate according to their particular expertise and the specific contribution they can make to a problem or issue, which itself may change over time. The danger with existing partnership arrangements, as many of our respondents told us, lies in them becoming an end in themselves, as distinct from being a means to an end. One interpretation of our findings is that they are pointing towards the need for a new and different approach; one that is consistent with a systems thinking perspective, which we outlined in Chapter Two.

We have emphasised the need for a systems perspective because building and managing partnerships is essential to it (De Savigny and Adam, 2009). A particular skill set is called for, which, without repeating much of what has been covered in earlier chapters, includes facilitating interdisciplinary meetings involving complex group dynamics and different perspectives. Typically, such skills are found in 'reticulists or boundary spanners' (Sullivan and Skelcher, 2002). Individuals falling into these categories are able to play a variety of roles that enable collaborations to work in ways that traditional meeting structures and procedures are unable to permit. Such skills need to be identified and nurtured – they do not just happen naturally. In particular, they demand lateral thinkers able to solve problems without being trapped in existing systems. 'Hard cooperation', insists Sennett in his discourse on the rituals, pleasures and politics of cooperation, requires 'dialogic skills', which include listening well, behaving tactfully, finding points of agreement and managing disagreement (Sennett, 2012, p 6).

The central point arising from systems thinking is the need for a different way of conceptualising and doing partnerships; one that embraces partnership working but that also advocates the adoption of a rather looser and less structured approach of the type mentioned earlier. Rather than there being a predetermined aim or purpose, the emphasis might be placed instead on getting started on some joint action without fully agreeing on aims – establishing what Huxham and Vangen (2005) call a 'working path'. Partnerships might benefit from becoming more exploratory, tentative and incremental, with both pre-set and emergent milestones identified. Importantly, the structural arrangements should be just sufficient enough to allow adequate exploration of the unknown. As Edmonstone (2010) argues, the approach to managing change in the NHS and elsewhere in the public sector has tended to proceed as if the problems being tackled are tame or critical or possibly complicated, but not complex.

However, as we have sought to demonstrate, the issues being confronted in public health are wicked ones, which demand a new and different approach to managing change. As a result, this will impact on both the nature and style of the partnerships needed to tackle such problems. While the early development of HWBs has been informed by such thinking and language, which has to be an advance on previous official discourses, there remain questions over how far in practice such entities will be allowed to work within a systems framework employing the dialogic skills considered by Sennett. The experience of Health Action Zones (HAZs) may be instructive here. Set up by New Labour in the late 1990s as bureaucracy-busting groups deliberately designed to be different and innovative, over their short history, they progressively became the most micro-managed and regulated part of the NHS architecture of any previous or subsequent partnership forms (Asthana et al, 2002; Barnes et al, 2005). Part of the change in atmosphere and style resulted from a change of health minister, and rather than being permitted to explore local issues in ways that involved risk-taking and promoting innovation, HAZs were progressively required to achieve national priorities. So, even with the best of intentions, it is quite possible to 'gang aft agley' and since changes of ministers is a regular feature of all governments, there can be no certainties about the fate of a particular initiative or guarantees that whatever they were introduced to achieve will endure.

In our view, and given what some of our respondents reported in interviews, and also, in part, drawing on the findings from the systematic literature review conducted for our study (Smith et al, 2009), there is a need to become less rigid and fixated on process, more open-ended and inclusive of diverse interests, especially those familiar with front-line work, and more focused on achieving ends that are emergent rather than predetermined. What our research also shows is that for all their positive features, at the time of the study, the arrangements of Local Strategic Partnerships (LSPs) and Local Area Agreements (LAAs) did not necessarily meet these requirements, but spawned a set of elaborate structures and procedures that, certainly in some cases, did not deliver what was required and might actually have served as a distraction from doing so.

The Total Place Pilots (TPPs), introduced by the Labour government towards the end of their period in office, so given insufficient time to prove themselves, were in one respect an acknowledgement, or admission, that existing partnerships were either not up to the job or were underachieving (HM Treasury and Department of Communities and Local Government, 2010). For instance, in some TPPs, innovative approaches exploring flexibilities were adopted to support local action to tackle chronic alcohol and drug misuse. However, cultural, organisational and capability barriers of the kind reported in our research posed major impediments to progress in many TPPs.

As mentioned, however, with the May 2010 election resulting in a Coalition government with quite different priorities, the initiative was given insufficient time to run its course, so it is not possible to be sure of their impact. What is true is that many of those giving evidence to the House of Commons Communities and Local Government Committee in its inquiry into health and local government proposed that future funding for public health should adopt a similar place-based approach to budgeting. And with the government's community-based budgets, although not as bold or extensive as TPP budgets, there is a glimmer of hope that such a solution may be possible. Such a form of budgeting would not only reinforce the need for effective partnerships, but also give them some clout.

At the same time, the desired redesign of services across organisational barriers is unlikely to be achieved through existing arrangements based on LSPs and LAAs, or even those emerging in some HWBs, which, although intended to be different, may revert to the default position. A host of cultural, structural and financial barriers need to be addressed in new ways so that resources (human and financial), instead of flowing through departmental silos, are allocated to problems or challenges affecting whole communities and places. Above all, what the discipline of the TPP approach requires is a whole-systems way of thinking about problem-solving, with key skills in appropriate leadership and partnership working in place.

A number of implications for partnerships and their future flow from the research presented in this book. A successful public health partnership is one which recognises that partnership working needs to be embedded in the culture from the bottom to the top in each partner organisation and between agencies. The partnership needs to be clear and realistic about its goals, to be adaptive and flexible, and to avoid a focus on structures; instead, being more holistic and organic in its approach to tackling 'wicked issues' in public health. This, in turn, allows for being innovative and flexible when confronting complex problems.

What this means in practice for partnerships, and to recap on the conclusions reached in Chapter Five, is the following set of precepts:

- Partnerships were deemed to be successful in their own terms when the policy processes were outcomes-focused, with joint delivery mechanisms, clear lines of accountability, the full engagement of relevant partners and careful monitoring. Conversely, less successful partnerships were deemed to be deficient in respect of these key features.

- An effective partnership was one where sharing information between agencies was assured alongside established information-sharing protocols in order to avoid duplication and encourage a coordinated approach.

- An effective partnership was one where all agencies were aware of their roles and responsibilities.

- A good partnership focused upon the needs of service users and ensured that they did not always have to give the same information to all other services with which they came into contact. The major benefit to service users, apart from a more seamless service, was acting as a signpost for other services they may need to access.

- Goodwill and trust between agencies was seen very much as the glue that held partnerships together, particularly on the front line. It was also the case that 'local champions' played a crucial role in partnerships, and they should be nurtured and supported.

- Different agency perspectives, it was believed, could lead to innovative solutions in tackling public health issues, from policy formulation to practical everyday contexts, by sharing the knowledge and expertise of partner agencies.

- A successful partnership was marked by pragmatism, flexibility and an organic quality, which got lost at higher levels, where the approach adopted was much more formal and governed by which structures were required to be put in place and which targets were to be met. The former qualities were very much in evidence with partnerships formed at the 'front line', which were much more flexible, holistic and organic in their approach to tackling public health issues and, as a result, were deemed more successful in pursuing their stated goals.

Although these are uncertain and difficult times for public health partnerships, they can succeed in the eyes of those running them, as our research and other work shows (Cameron and Lart, 2003; Dowling et al, 2004), although their impact on public health outcomes is thus far limited and hard to assess. The partnerships that do succeed possess all, or most, of the features and ingredients highlighted earlier. Putting in place the softer aspects around relationships and dialogic skills is also central to the success of partnerships and to ensuring that they do not become over-engineered and bureaucratic. As we suggested earlier, a degree of messiness may be no bad thing to include in the mix of ingredients that go to make for an effective partnership. Mess is about flexibility, variation, inconsistency and the unexpected (Abrahamson and Freedman, 2006). Of course, this makes it impossible and self-defeating to extract the rules and principles that expose the secrets of messy organisations and leaders. However, a weakness, sometimes failing, of LSPs and other previous partnership forms is that too much attention has sometimes been focused on structure without attending to issues of membership and the skills needed, including high emotional intelligence and political astuteness. In the new and unpredictable world we have entered, such skills and attributes are going to become ever-more crucial and count for more than simply trying to get the structures right.

HWBs 'will bring together the key NHS, public health and social care leaders in each local authority area to work in partnership ... which would also increase the local democratic legitimacy of NHS commissioning decisions' (Secretary of State for Health, 2010c, p 97, para 5.5). They cannot afford to focus exclusively on structural questions without attending to these other critical matters. If structure becomes their central focus, then HWBs will surely fail, as previous partnerships have often done. However, perhaps the greatest risk is that establishing HWBs once again means public health partnerships having to start largely from scratch, with the inevitable loss of corporate memory, and having to rebuild relationships and networks at a time when there are limited resources to do so and not much time to prove themselves and make an impact. Conceivably, such factors could herald a new dawn for partnership working that is less encumbered by the past or cluttered with previous organisational forms that may no longer be fit for purpose. However, to seize these opportunities means avoiding a path-dependent approach, whereby the focus is on continuing to do what has always been done simply because it has always been done that way.

Finally, throughout this exploration of partnerships, we have stressed the importance of overall policy alignment and coherence. This is because all the evidence suggests that what can be achieved locally will be limited at best, and possibly fail at worst, unless there is effective synergy and coherence across the policy pathway from top to bottom (Parker et al, 2010). An overbearing top-down policy approach, combined with mixed and even contradictory messages coming from different bodies at the centre, can have a detrimental effect on partnerships and on the morale of those working in them. The Coalition government seems to have grasped this weakness with its emphasis on localism, but its words and its actions have not always been joined-up themselves and there is a concern that despite the public rhetoric surrounding localism, there remains a strong pull to the centre behind the façade. It seems likely that, for a number of reasons, but perhaps principally because a general election will take place in 2015, such pressures, with all the consequences likely to flow from them, can only grow in intensity.

Traditionally, governments have sought to diffuse blame while centralising credit, and although that principle is likely to be upheld by the present government, there remains a worry that localism might not be good news for central government if it gets the blame for too much diversity and variation of the kind that erupts from time to time over postcode rationing in respect of health care and the patchy prescribing of particular high-cost drugs. If the public experience of localism is a negative one, then it will be central government that is likely to get the blame.

Last word

To conclude, as noted earlier, we cannot yet judge the potential effectiveness of the Coalition government's public health reforms, which have partnerships as one of their core elements, but one thing is clear: effective partnership working will be the key to any success the government may seek to claim. A problem will arise, as so often in the past, if governments simply subscribe to the triumph of hope over experience. We mean by this that too often policy changes rely heavily on hope and too little on learning the lessons from experience (Edwards, 2010). Such faith-based policy can be no substitute for proper analysis of what will enable public health partnerships to succeed. We have drawn attention to a research-based literature reinforcing the importance of culture, values, processes and systems over structure. In that famous phrase: 'culture eats structure for breakfast any day'. In leaving the new partnership forms in the shape of HWBs with a single last thought that seeks to distil much of what has been presented in the preceding chapters, we can think of none better.

References

Abrahamson, E. and Freedman, D.H. (2006) *A perfect mess: the hidden benefits of disorder*, London: Weidenfeld and Nicolson.

Acheson, D. (1998) *Public health in England. The report of the committee of inquiry into the future development of the public health function*, London: HMSO.

*Arora, S., Davies, A. and Thompson, S. (1999) *Developing health improvement programmes: lessons from the first year*, London: The King's Fund.

*Arora, S., Davies, A. and Thompson, S. (2000) 'Developing health improvement programmes: challenges for a new millennium', *Journal of Inter-professional Care*, vol 14, no 1, pp 9–18.

Asthana, S., Richardson, S. and Halliday, J. (2002) 'Partnership working in public policy provision: a framework for evaluation', *Social Policy and Administration*, vol 36, pp 780–95.

Audit Commission (1998) *A fruitful partnership: effective partnership working*, London: Audit Commission.

Audit Commission (2005) *Governing partnerships: bridging the accountability gap*, London: Audit Commission.

Audit Commission (2009) *Means to an end: joint financing across health and social care*, London: Audit Commission.

Audit Commission, Care Quality Commission, HM Inspectorate of Constabulary, HM Inspectorate of Prisons, HM Inspectorate of Probation and Ofsted (2009) *Comprehensive area assessment: a guide to the new framework*, London: Audit Commission.

Australian Public Service Commission (2007) *Tackling wicked problems: a public policy perspective*, Canberra: Commonwealth of Australia.

Bacon, N. and Samuel, P. (2012) *Partnership in NHS Scotland 1999–2011*, London: Economic and Social Research Council.

Balloch, S. and Taylor, M. (2001a) 'Conclusion', in S. Balloch and M. Taylor (eds) *Partnership working: policy and practice*, Bristol: The Policy Press.

Balloch, S. and Taylor, M. (2001b) 'Introduction', in S. Balloch and M. Taylor (eds) *Partnership working: policy and practice*, Bristol: The Policy Press.

Barnes, M., Bauld, L., Benzeval, M., Judge, K., Mackenzie, M. and Sullivan, H. (2005) *Health action zones: partnerships for health equity*, London: Routledge.

*Bauld, L., Judge, K., Lawson, L., Mackenzie, M., Mackinnon, J. and Truman, J. (2001) *Health Action Zones in transition: progress in 2000*, Glasgow: Health Promotion Policy Unit, University of Glasgow.

*Bauld, L., Judge K., Barnes, M., Benzeval, M., Mackenzie, M. and Sullivan, H. (2005a) 'Promoting social change: the experience of Health Action Zones in England', *Journal of Social Policy*, vol 34, pp 427–45.

*Bauld, L., Sullivan, H., Judge, K. and Mackinnon, J. (2005b) 'Assessing the impact of Health Action Zones', in M. Barnes, L. Bauld, M. Benzeval, K. Judge, M. Mackenzie and H. Sullivan (eds) *Health Action Zones: partnerships for health equity*, London: Routledge, pp 157–84.

Bentley, C. (2013) 'Public health and local authorities, written submission', in House of Commons Communities and Local Government Committee *The role of local authorities in health issues. Eighth report of session 2012–13*, HC 694, Ev 15–65, London: The Stationery Office.

*Benzeval, M. (2003) *The final report of the Tackling Inequalities in Health module*, London: Queen Mary, University of London.

*Benzeval, M. and Meth, F. (2002) *Health inequalities: a priority at a crossroads – the final report to the Department of Health*, London: Department of Health.

*Bhatti, S., Cuthburt, V. and Lunt, J. (2002) 'The pampering gang project', in L. Bauld and K. Judge (eds) *Learning from Health Action Zones*, Chichester: Aeneas Press, pp 251–62.

**Blackman, T., Wistow, J. and Byrne, D. (2011) 'Towards a new understanding of how local action can effectively address health inequalities', report for the National Institute for Health Research Service Delivery and Organisation Programme.

*Bonner, L. (2003) 'Using theory-based evaluation to build evidence-based health and social care policy and practice', *Critical Public Health*, vol 13, no 1, pp 77–92.

Boyle, S. (2011) 'United Kingdom (England) health system review', *Health Systems in Transition*, vol 13, no 1, pp 1–486, Copenhagen: European Observatory on Health Systems and Policies.

Buck, D. and Frosini, F. (2012) *Clustering of unhealthy behaviours over time: implications for policy and practice*, London: The King's Fund.

*Burton, S. and Diaz de Leon, D. (2002) 'An evaluation of benefits advice in primary care: Camden and Islington Health Action Zone', in L. Bauld and K. Judge (eds) *Learning from Health Action Zones*, Chichester: Aeneas Press, pp 241–50.

Butland, B., Jebb, S., Kopelman, P., McPherson, K., Thomas, S., Mardell, J. and Parry, V. (2007) *Tackling obesities: future choices – project report*, commissioned by the UK Government's Foresight Programme, Government Office for Science, London: The Stationery Office. Available at: http://www.foresight.gov.uk/OurWork/ActiveProjects/Obesity/Obesity.asp

Cabinet Office (1999) *Modernising government*, London: The Stationery Office.

*Cameron, A. and Lart, R. (2003) 'Factors promoting and obstacles hindering joint working: a systematic review of the research evidence', *Journal of Integrated Care*, vol 11, no 2, pp 9–17.

Carlisle, S. (2001) 'Inequalities in health: contested explanations, shifting discourses and ambiguous policies', *Critical Public Health*, vol 11, no 3, pp 267–81.

Chapman J. (2004) *System failure: why governments must learn to think differently* (2nd edn), London: Demos.

Churchill, N. (ed) (2012) *Getting started: prospects for Health and Wellbeing Boards*, London: The Smith Institute.

Clarke, E. and Glendinning, C. (2002) 'Partnership and the remaking of welfare governance', in C. Glendinning, M. Powell and K. Rummery (eds) *Partnerships, New Labour and the governance of welfare*, Bristol: The Policy Press.

*Cole, M. (2003) 'The Health Action Zone initiative: lessons from Plymouth', *Local Government Studies*, vol 29, no 3, pp 99–117.

Cooper, Z., Gibbons, S., Jones, S. and McGuire, A. (2011) 'Does hospital competition save lives? Evidence from the English NHS patient choice reforms', *Economic Journal*, vol 121, pp 228–60.

*CRESR (Centre for Regional Economic and Social Research) (2005) *New Deal for Communities 2001–2005: an interim evaluation*, London: ODPM Publications.

DCLG (Department for Communities and Local Government) (2006) *Strong and prosperous communities: the local government White Paper*, London: Department for Communities and Local Government.

Deeks, J., Dinnes, J., D'Amico, R., Sowde, A.J., Sakarovitch, C., Song, F., Petticrew, M. and Altman, D.G. (2003) 'Evaluating non-randomised intervention studies', *Health Technology Assessment*, vol 7, no 27, pp 1–173.

Department of Health (2001) *The report of the Chief Medical Officer's project to strengthen the public health function*, London: Department of Health.

Department of Health (2008a) *Tackling health inequalities: 2007 status report on programme for action*, London: Department of Health.

Department of Health (2008b) *Health inequalities: progress and next steps*, London: Department of Health.

Department of Health (2010) *Review of the regulation of public health professionals*, London: Department of Health.

Department of Health (2011a) *Public health in local government factsheets*, London: Department of Health.

Department of Health (2011b) *Public Health England's operating model factsheets*, London: Department of Health.

Department of Health (2012a) *The mandate: a mandate from the government to the NHS Commissioning Board: April 2013 to March 2015*, London: Department of Health.

Department of Health (2012b) *Structure of Public Health England, factsheet*, London: Department of Health.

Department of Health (2012c) *Healthy lives, healthy people: improving outcomes and supporting transparency*, London: Department of Health.

Department of Health (2013a) *Government response to the House of Commons Communities and Local Government Committee Eighth Report of Session 2012–13: The role of local authorities in health issues*, Cm 8638, London: The Stationery Office.

Department of Health (2013b) *Living well for longer: a call to action to reduce avoidable premature mortality*, London: Department of Health.

Department of Health (2013c) *Refreshing the mandate to NHS England: 2014–2015*, Consultation, London: Department of Health.

Department of Health and Department for Communities and Local Government (2013) 'Written submission', in House of Commons Communities and Local Government Committee, *The role of local authorities in health issues*, Eighth Report of Session 2012–13, HC 694, Ev 165, London: The Stationery Office.

De Savigny, D. and Adam, T. (eds) (2009) *Systems thinking for health systems strengthening*, Geneva: Alliance for Health Policy and System Research, World Health Organization.

Dickinson, H. (2007) 'Evaluating the outcomes of health and social care partnerships: the POET approach', *Research, Policy and Planning*, vol 25, nos 2/3, pp 79–92.

Dickinson, H. (2008) *Evaluating outcomes in health and social care*, Bristol: The Policy Press.

Dickinson, H. and Glasby, J. (2010) 'Why partnership working doesn't work: pitfalls, problems and possibilities in English health and social care', *Public Management Review*, vol 12, no 6, pp 811–28.

Dixon-Woods, M., Cavers, D., Agarwal, S., Annandale, E., Arthur, A., Harvey, J., Hsu, R., Katbamna, S., Olsen, R., Smith, L., Riley, R. and Sutton, A.J. (2006) 'Conducting a critical interpretive synthesis of the literature on access to healthcare by vulnerable groups', *BMC Medical Research Methodology*, vol 6, no 35, pp 1–13.

Douglas, A. (2009) *Partnership working*, London: Routledge.

Dowling, B., Powell, M. and Glendinning, C. (2004) 'Conceptualising successful partnerships', *Health and Social Care in the Community*, vol 12, no 4, pp 309–17.

*Durham University (2008) 'The Smoke-Free North East Advisory Panel: an ethnographic analysis of one-on-one relationships in a public health partnership', unpublished paper.

Edmonstone, J. (2010) 'A new approach to project managing change', *British Journal of Healthcare Management*, vol 16, no 5, pp 225–30.

Edwards, N. (2010) *The triumph of hope over experience: lessons from the history of reorganisation*, London: NHS Confederation.

Egan, M., Bambra, C., Petticrew, M., Whitehead, M., Thomas, S. and Thompson, H.(2007) 'The psychosocial and health effects of work place reorganisation. 1. A systematic review of organisational-level interventions that aim to increase employee control', *Journal of Epidemiology & Community Health*, vol 61, no 11, pp 945–54.

Elmore, R.F. (1979) 'Backward mapping: implementation research and policy decisions', *Political Science Quarterly*, vol 94, no 4, pp 601–16.

Elson, T. (1999) 'Public health and local government', in S. Griffiths and D.J. Hunter (eds) *Perspectives in public health*, Oxford: Radcliffe Medical Press.

Elson, T. (2004) 'Why public health must become a core part of council agendas', in K. Skinner (ed) *Community leadership and public health: the role of local authorities*, London: The Smith Institute.

*Evans, D. and Killoran, A. (2000) 'Tackling health inequalities through partnership working: learning from a realistic evaluation', *Critical Public Health*, vol 10, no 2, pp 125–40.

Evans, D. and Knight, T. (2006) *'There was no plan!' The origins and development of multi-disciplinary public health in the UK*, witness seminar, Bristol: University of the West of England.

Exworthy, M. and Hunter, D.J. (2011) 'The challenge of joined-up government in tackling health inequalities', *International Journal of Public Administration*, vol 34, no 4, pp 201–12.

Figueras, J., McKee, M., Lessof, S., Durhan, A. and Menabde, N. (2008) *Health systems, health and wealth: assessing the case for investing in health systems*, Copenhagen: WHO.

Francis, R. (2013) *Report of the Mid Staffordshire NHS Foundation Trust public inquiry*, London: The Stationery Office.

*Freeman, T. and Peck, E. (2006) 'Evaluating partnerships: a case study of integrated specialist mental health services', *Health and Social Care in the Community*, vol 14, no 5, pp 408–17.

Gash, T., Panchamia, N., Sims, S. and Hotson, L. (2013) *Making public service markets work*, London: Institute for Government.

Gaynor, M., Proppper, C. and Seller, S. (2012) 'Free to choose? Reform and demand response in the English National Health Service'. Available at: www.nber.org/papers/w18574

*Geller, R. (2001) 'The first year of Health Improvement Programmes; views from Directors of Public Health', *Journal of Public Health Medicine*, vol 23, no 1, pp 57–64.

Gilmore, A.B. (2001) 'Joint working, reality or rhetoric?', *Journal of Public Health Medicine*, vol 23, no 1, pp 5–6.

Glasby, J. and Dickinson, H. (2008) *Partnership working in health and social care*, Bristol: The Policy Press.

*Glendinning, C., Coleman, A., Shipman, C. and Malbon, G. (2001) 'Primary care groups: progress in partnerships', *British Medical Journal*, vol 323, pp 28–31.

Glendinning, C., Dowling, B. and Powell, M. (2005a) 'Partnerships between health and social care under "New Labour": smoke without fire? A review of policy and evidence', *Evidence & Policy: A Journal of Research, Debate and Practice*, vol 1, no 3, pp 365–82.

Glendinning, C., Hudson, B. and Means, R. (2005b) 'Under strain? Exploring the troubled relationship between health and social care', *Public Money and Management*, vol 25, no 4, pp 245–51.

Gorsky, M. (2007) 'Local leadership in public health: the role of the Medical Officer of Health in Britain, 1872–1974', *Journal of Epidemiology and Community Health*, vol 61, no 6, pp 468–72.

Grady, M. (2013) 'Health inequity, partnership and the role of local government, written submission', in House of Commons Communities and Local Government Committee, *The role of local authorities in health issues. Eighth report of session 2012–13*, HC 694, Ev 146–9, London: The Stationery Office.

Grady, M. and Goldblatt, P. (eds) (2012) *Addressing the social determinants of health: the urban dimension and the role of local government*, Copenhagen: World Health Organization.

Graham, H. (2010) 'Where is the future in public health?', *The Milbank Quarterly*, vol 88, no 2, pp 149–68.

Gray, B. (1989) *Collaborating: finding common ground for multiparty problems*, San Francisco, CA: Josey Bass.

Griffiths, S., Jewell, T. and Donnelly, P. (2005) 'Public health in practice: the three domains of public health', *Public Health*, vol 119, no 10, pp 907–13.

Grint, K. (2010) *Purpose, power, knowledge, time and space: total pilot final research report*, London: Local Government Leadership and Warwick Business School.

*Halliday, J. and Asthana, S. (2005) 'Policy at the margins: developing community capacity in a rural Health Action Zone', *Area*, vol 37, pp 180–8.

Hannaway, C., Plsek, P. and Hunter, D.J. (2007) 'Developing leadership and management for health', in D.J. Hunter (ed) *Managing for health*, London: Routledge, pp 148–73.

Hardy, B., Hudson, B. and Waddington, E. (2003) *Assessing strategic partnership: the partnership assessment tool*, London: ODPM.

Hastings, G. (2012) 'Why corporate power is a public health priority', *British Medical Journal*, vol 345, e5124.

Healthcare Commission and Audit Commission (2008) *Are we choosing health? The impact of policy on the delivery of health improvement programmes and services*, London: Commission for Healthcare Audit and Inspection.

*Health Development Agency (2005) *The Healthier Communities Shared Priority Project: learning from the pathfinder authorities*, London: HDA.

Hicks, N. (2013) *Oral evidence taken before the CLG, 26 November 2012*, London: The Stationery Office.

*Hills, D., Elliott, E., Kowarzik, U., Sullivan, F., Stern, E., Platt, S., Boydell, L., Popay, J., Williams, G., Petticrew, M., McGregor, E., Russell, S., Wilkinson, E., Rugkasa, J., Gibson, M. and McDaid, D. (2007) *The evaluation of the Big Lottery Fund Healthy Living Centres programme: final report – January 2007*, London: Big Lottery Fund.

HM Treasury and Department for Communities and Local Government (2010) *Total Place: a whole area approach to public services*, London: HM Treasury and DCLG.

House of Commons Communities and Local Government Committee (2013) *The role of local authorities in health issues. Eighth report of session 2012–13*, HC 694, London: The Stationery Office.

House of Commons Health Committee (2011) *Public health. Twelfth report of session 2010–12. Volume I: report*, HC 1048-I, London: The Stationery Office.

Hudson, B. (2004) 'Analysing network partnerships: Benson re-visited', *Public Management Review*, vol 6, no 1, pp 75–94.

Hudson, B., Hardy, B., Henwood, M. and Wistow, G. (1999) 'In pursuit of inter-agency collaboration in the public sector', *Public Management: An International Journal of Research and Theory*, vol 1, no 2, pp 235–60.

Hughes, L. (2013) 'Written submission', in House of Commons Communities and Local Government Committee, *The role of local authorities in health issues. Eighth report of session 2012–13*, HC 694, Ev 124–6, London: The Stationery Office.

Humphries, R. (2013) *How are Health and Wellbeing Boards shaping up to their new responsibilities?*, The King's Fund Blog, London: The King's Fund.

Humphries, R. and Gregory, S. (2010) *Place-based approaches and the NHS: lessons from Total Place*, London: The King's Fund.

Humphries, R., Galea, A., Sonola, L. and Mundle, C. (2012) *Health and Wellbeing Boards: system leaders or talking shops?*, London: The King's Fund.

Hunter, D.J. (2003) *Public health policy*, Cambridge: Polity.

Hunter, D.J. (2005) 'Choosing or losing health?', *Journal of Epidemiology and Community Health*, vol 59, no 12, pp 1010–12.

Hunter, D.J. (ed) (2007a) *Managing for health*, London: Routledge.

Hunter, D.J. (2007b) *Learning from Healthy Living Centres: the changing policy context, Big Lottery Fund policy commentary – issue 1*, London: Big Lottery Fund.

Hunter, D.J. (2008a) 'Introduction and background', in D.J. Hunter (ed) *Perspectives on Joint Director of Public Health appointments*, London: Improvement and Development Agency.

Hunter, D.J. (2008b) *The health debate*, Bristol: The Policy Press.

Hunter, D.J. (2011) 'Change of government: one more big bang health care reform in England's National Health Service', *International Journal of Health Services*, vol 41, no 1, pp 159–74.

Hunter, D.J., Marks, L. and Smith, K.E. (2010) *The public health system in England*, Bristol: The Policy Press.

Huxham, C. (2003) 'Theorizing collaboration practice', *Public Management Review*, vol 5, no 3, pp 401–23.

Huxham, C. and Vangen, S. (2000) 'What makes partnership work?', in S. Osborne (ed) *Public–Private Partnerships*, London: Routledge.

Huxham, C. and Vangen, S. (2005) *Managing to collaborate: the theory and practice of collaborative advantage*, Abingdon: Routledge.

Huxham, C., Vangen, S. and Eden, C. (2000) 'The challenge of collaborative governance', *Public Management: An International Journal of Research and Theory*, vol 2, no 3, pp 337–58.

IDeA (Improvement and Development Agency) (2007) *Healthy communities peer review. Guidance for authorities*, London: IDeA, pp 20–38.

IOM (Institute of Medicine) (2003) *The future of the public's health in the 21st century*, Washington, DC: The National Academies Press.

*Jacobs, B., Mulroy, S. and Sime, C. (2002) 'Theories of chance and community involvement in North Staffordshire Health Action Zone', in L. Bauld and K. Judge (eds) *Learning from Health Action Zones*, Chichester: Aeneas, pp 139–48.

Jacobson, B., Smith, A. and Whitehead, M. (1991) *The nation's health: a strategy for the 1990s*, London: King Edward's Hospital Fund for London.

*Kane, B. (2002) 'Social capital, health and economy in South Yorkshire coalfield communities', in L. Bauld and K. Judge (eds) *Learning from Health Action Zones*, Chichester: Aeneas Press, pp 187–98.

Keohane, N. and Smith, G. (2010) *Greater than the sum of its parts: Total Place and the future shape of public services*, London: New Local Government Network.

Labour Party (1997) *New Labour because Britain deserves better, The Labour Party Manifesto*, London: Labour Party.

Lang, T. and Rayner, G. (2012) 'Ecological public health: the 21st century's big idea?', *British Medical Journal*, vol 345, e5466.

Leadbeater, C. (1999) *Living on thin air: the new economy*, London: Viking.

Lewis, J. (1986) *What price community medicine? The philosophy, practice and politics of public health since 1919*, Brighton: Wheatsheaf.

Ling, T. (2002) 'Delivering joined-up government in the UK: dimensions, issues and problems', *Public Administration*, vol 80, no 4, pp 615–42.

Litvack, J., Ahmad, J. and Bird, R. (1998) *Rethinking decentralisation in developing countries*, Washington, DC: World Bank.

Local Government Centre (2007) 'Themes and trends in signed-off round 2 Local Area Agreements', Institute of Governance and public Management, Warwick Business School, University of Warwick.

Longley, M., Riley, N., Davies, P. and Hernandez-Quevedo, C. (2012) 'United Kingdom (Wales) health system review', *Health Systems in Transition*, vol 14, no 11, pp 1–84, Copenhagen: European Observatory on Health Systems and Policies.

Lowndes, V. and Skelcher, C. (1998) 'The dynamics of multi-organisational partnerships: an analysis of changing modes of governance', *Public Administration*, vol 76, Summer, pp 313–33.

Lowndes, V. and Sullivan, H. (2004) 'Like a horse and carriage or a fish on a bicycle: how well do local partnerships and public participation go together?', *Local Government Studies*, vol 30, no 1, pp 51–73.

Lyons, M. (2007) *Lyons Inquiry into Local Government – Place-shaping: a shared ambition for the future of local government*, London: The Stationery Office.

McCarthy, B. (2013) *Government consultation on the mandate*, Board Paper, NHS England.

McDonald, I. (2005) 'Theorising partnerships: governance, communicative action and sport policy', *Journal of Social Policy*, vol 34, no 4, pp 579–600.

McKee, M., Hurst, C., Aldridge, R.W., Paine, R., Mindell, J.S., Wolfe, I. and Holland, W.W. (2011) 'Public health in England: an option for the way forward', *The Lancet*, vol 378, no 9980, pp 536–9.

*Mackenzie, M., Lawson, L., Mackinnon, J., Meth, F. and Truman, J. (2003) *National evaluation of Health Action Zones – the integrated case studies: a move toward whole systems change*, Glasgow: University of Glasgow.

Mackintosh, M. (1993) 'Partnership: issues of policy and negotiation', *Local Economy*, vol 7, no 3, pp 210–24.

**Marks, L., Cave, S., Hunter, D.J., Mason, J., Peckham, S., Wallace, A., Mason, A., Weatherly, H. and Melvin, K. (2011) *Public health governance and primary care delivery: a triangulated study. Final report*, Southampton: NIHR Service Delivery and Organisation programme.

Marks, L., Hunter, D.J. and Alderslade, R. (2011) *Strengthening public health capacity and services in Europe: a concept paper*, Copenhagen: WHO.

*Matka, E., Barnes, M. and Sullivan, H. (2002) 'Health Action Zones: creating alliances to achieve change', *Policy Studies Journal*, vol 23, pp 92–106.

Milburn, A. (2000) 'A healthier nation and a healthier economy: the contribution of a modern NHS', LSE Health Annual Lecture, 8 March, London.

National Audit Office (2010a) *Reorganising central government*, London: The Stationery Office.

National Audit Office (2010b) *Tackling inequalities in life expectancy in areas with the worst health and deprivation*, London: The Stationery Office.

National Leadership and Innovation Agency for Healthcare (2009) *Getting collaboration to work in Wales: lessons from the NHS and its partners*, Cardiff: NLIAH.

NHS Future Forum (2012) *The NHS's role in the public's health: a report for the NHS Future Forum*, London: Department of Health.

ODPM (Office of the Deputy Prime Minister) (2005) *Evaluation of Local Strategic Partnerships: interim report*, London: ODPM.

O'Neill, J., McGregor, P. and Merkur, S. (2012) 'United Kingdom (Northern Ireland) health system review', *Health Systems in Transition*, vol 14, no 10, pp 1–91, Copenhagen: European Observatory on Health Systems and Policies.

Organisation for Economic Co-operation and Development (1990) *Partnerships for rural development*, Paris: OECD.

Parker, S., Paun, A., McClory, J. and Blatchford, K. (2010) *Shaping up: a Whitehall for the future*, London: Institute for Government.

Penhale, B., Perkins, N., Pinkney, L., Reid, D., Hussein, S. and Manthorpe, J. (2007) 'Partnership and regulation in adult protection. The effectiveness of multi-agency working and the regulatory framework in adult protection. Final report'. Available at: http://www.prap.group.shef.ac.uk/ (accessed November 2012).

Pollitt, C. (2003) *The essential public manager*, Maidenhead: Open University Press.

Pollock, A., Macfarlane, A., Kirkwood, G., Majeed, F.A., Greener, I., Morelli, C., Boyle, S., Mellett, H., Godden, S., Price, D. and Brhlikova, P. (2011) 'No evidence that patient choice saves lives', *Lancet*, vol 378, pp 2057–60.

Popay, J., Whitehead, M. and Hunter, D.J. (2010) 'Injustice is killing people on a large scale – but what is to be done about it?', *Journal of Public Health*, vol 32, no 2, pp 150–6.

Powell, M. and Dowling, B. (2006) 'New Labour's partnerships: comparing conceptual models with existing forms', *Social Policy and Society*, vol 5, no 2, pp 305–14.

Powell, M. and Exworthy, M. (2001) 'Joined-up solutions to address health inequalities: analysing policy, process and resource streams', *Public Money and Management*, January–March.

Powell, M. and Exworthy, M. (2002) 'Partnerships, quasi-networks and social policy', in C. Glendinning, M. Powell and K. Rummery (eds) *Partnerships, New Labour and the governance of welfare*, Bristol: The Policy Press.

Powell, M. and Glendinning, C. (2002) 'Introduction', in C. Glendinning, M. Powell and K. Rummery (eds) *Partnerships, New Labour and the governance of welfare*, Bristol: The Policy Press.

*Powell, M., Exworthy, M. and Berney, L. (2001) 'Playing the game of partnership', in R. Sykes, C. Bochel and N. Ellison (eds) *Social policy review 13, developments and debates: 2000–2001*, Bristol: The Policy Press.

Powell, W. (1991) 'Neither market nor hierarchy: Network forms of organisation', in G. Thompson, J. Frances, R. Levacic and J. Mitchell (eds) *Markets, hierarchies and networks: the co-ordination of social life*, London: SAGE.

Public Health Resource Unit (2006) 'Critical Appraisal Skills Programme (CASP). 10 questions to help you make sense of qualitative research'. Available at: http://www.phru.nhs.uk/Pages/PHD/resources.htm (accessed 7 December 2007).

Ranade, W. and Hudson, B. (2003) 'Conceptual issues in inter-agency collaboration', *Local Government Studies*, vol 29, no 3, pp 32–50.

Rees, R., Kavanagh, J., Harden, A., Shepherd, J., Brunton, G., Oliver, S. and Oakley, A. (2006) 'Young people and physical activity: a systematic review matching their views to effective interventions', *Health Education Research*, vol 21, no 6, pp 806–25.

Rittel, H.W.J. and Webber, M.M. (1973) 'Dilemmas in a general theory of planning', *Policy Sciences*, vol 4, no 2, pp 155–69.

Rogers, D. (2012) 'Developing relationships – the role of local government', in N. Churchill (ed) *Getting started: prospects for Health and Wellbeing Boards*, London: The Smith Institute.

Royal College of Nursing (2013) 'Written submission', in House of Commons Communities and Local Government Committee, *The role of local authorities in health issues. Eighth report of session 2012–13*, HC 694, Ev 104–08, London: The Stationery Office.

Royal Town Planning Institute (2013) 'Written submission', in House of Commons Communities and Local Government Committee, *The role of local authorities in health issues. Eighth report of session 2012–13*, HC 694, Ev 111–14, London: The Stationery Office.

Rummery, K. (2002) 'Towards a theory of welfare partnerships', in C. Glendinning, M. Powell and K. Rummery (eds) *Partnerships, New Labour and the governance of welfare*, Bristol: The Policy Press.

Scally, G. (2013a) 'Written submission', in House of Commons Communities and Local Government Committee, *The role of local authorities in health issues. Eighth report of session 2012–13*, HC 694, Ev 98–9, London: The Stationery Office.

Scally, G. (2013b) *Oral evidence taken before the CLG, 26 November 2012*, London: The Stationery Office.

Secretary of State for Health (1999) *Saving lives: our healthier nation*, Cm 4386, London: The Stationery Office.

Secretary of State for Health (2004) *Choosing health: making healthy choices easier*, Cm 6374, London: The Stationery Office.

Secretary of State for Health (2010a) *Equity and excellence: liberating the NHS*, Cm 7881, London: Department of Health.

Secretary of State for Health (2010b) *Healthy lives, healthy people: our strategy for public health in England*, Cm 7985, London: HM Government.

Secretary of State for Health (2010c) *Liberating the NHS: legislative framework and next steps*, Cm 7993, London: Department of Health.

Secretary of State for Health (2012) *Government response to the House of Commons Health Committee report on public health (twelfth report of session 2010–12)*, Cm 8290, London: Department of Health.

Seddon, J. (2008) *Systems thinking in the public sector*, Axminster: Triarchy Press.

Sennett, R. (2006) *The culture of the new capitalism*, London: Yale University Press.

Sennett, R. (2012) *Together: the rituals, pleasures and politics of cooperation*, London: Allen Lane.

Simon, H.A. (1957) *Administrative behaviour*, New York, NY: Free Press.

Smith, K.E., Hunter, D.J., Blackman, T., Elliott, E., Greene, A., Harrington, B.E., Marks, L., McKee, L. and Williams, G.H. (2008) 'Diversity or convergence? Health inequalities and policy in a devolved Britain', *Critical Social Policy*, vol 29, no 2, pp 216–42.

Smith, K., Bambra, C., Joyce, K.E., Perkins, N., Hunter, D.J. and Blenkinsopp, E. (2009) 'Partners in health? A systematic review of the impact of organizational partnerships on public health outcomes in England between 1997 and 2008', *Journal of Public Health*, vol 31, no 2, pp 210–21. Available at: http://jpubhealth.oxfordjournals.org/cgi/reprint/fdp002

★Speller, V. (1999) *Promoting community health: developing the role of local government*, London: Health Education Authority.

★Stafford, M., Nazroo, J., Popay, J.M. and Whitehead, M. (2008) 'Tackling inequalities in health: evaluating the New Deal for Communities initiative', *Journal of Epidemiology and Community Health*, vol 62, pp 298–304.

Stahl, T., Wismar, M., Ollilia, E., Lahtinen, E. and Leppo, K. (eds) (2006) *Health in all policies: prospects and potentials*, Helsinki: Finnish Ministry of Health and Social Affairs and Health and European Observatory on Health Systems and Policies. Available at: www.euro.who.int/document/E89260.pdf

Steel, D. and Cylus, J. (2012) 'United Kingdom (Scotland) Health system review', *Health Systems in Transition*, vol 14, no 9, pp 1–150, Copenhagen, European Observatory on Health Systems and Policies.

Stewart, J. (1998) 'Advance or retreat: from the traditions of public administration to the new public management and beyond', *Public Policy and Administration*, vol 13, no 4, pp 12–27.

Sullivan, H. and Skelcher, C. (2002) *Working across boundaries: collaboration in public services*, Basingstoke: Palgrave.

★Sullivan, H., Barnes, M. and Matka, E. (2002) 'Building collaborative capacity through theories of change', *Evaluation*, vol 8, pp 205–26.

*Sullivan, H., Judge, K. and Sewel, K. (2004) '"In the eye of the beholder": perceptions of local impact in English Health Action Zones', *Social Science & Medicine*, vol 59, pp 1603–12.

*Sullivan, H., Barnes, M. and Matka, E. (2005) 'Building capacity for collaboration', in M. Barnes, L. Bauld, M. Benzeval, K. Judge, M. Mackenzie and H. Sullivan (eds) *Health Action Zones: partnerships for health equity*, London: Routledge, pp 87–114.

Taylor-Gooby, P. and Stoker, G. (2011) 'The Coalition programme: a new vision for Britain or politics as usual?', *The Political Quarterly*, vol 82, no 1, pp 4–15.

**Taylor-Robinson, D.C., Lloyd-Williams, F., Orton, L., Moonan, M., O'Flaherty, M. and Capewell, S. (2012) 'Barriers to partnership working in public health: a qualitative study', *PLoS ONE*, vol 7, no 1, e29536, doi:10.1371/journal.pone.0029536.

*TCRU (Thomas Coram Research Unit) and NFER (National Foundation for Educational Research) (2004) *Evaluation of the impact of the National Healthy School Standard*, London: Department of Health.

UK Healthy Cities Network (2013) 'Written submission', in House of Commons Communities and Local Government Committee, *The role of local authorities in health issues*, Eighth report of session 2012–13, HC 694, vol 11, Ev W19.

Walshe, K. (2010) 'Reorganisation of the NHS in England', *British Medical Journal*, vol 341, c3790, doi: 10.1136/bmj.c3790.

Wanless, D. (2002) *Securing our future health: taking a long-term view, final report*, London: HM Treasury.

Wanless, D. (2004) *Securing good health for the whole population, final report*, London: Department of Health.

Wanless, D., Appleby, J., Harrison, A. and Patel, D. (2007) *Our future health secured? A review of NHS funding and performance*, London: The Kings Fund.

Wilding, K. (2010) 'Voluntary organisations and the recession', *Voluntary Sector Review*, vol 1, no 1, pp 97–101.

Wildridge, V., Childs, S., Cawthra, L. and Madge, B. (2004) 'How to create successful partnerships – a review of the literature', *Health Information and Libraries Journal*, vol 21, no 3, pp 3–19.

Williams, P. and Sullivan, H. (2009) 'Faces of integration', *International Journal of Integrated Care*, 9, 22 December

Williams, P. and Sullivan, H. (2010) 'Despite all we know about collaborative working, why do we still get it wrong?', *Journal of Integrated Care*, vol 18, no 4, pp 4–15.

WHO (World Health Organization) (2008) *The Tallinn Charter: health systems for health and wealth*, Copenhagen: WHO Europe.

WHO (2012) *Governance for health in the 21st century*, Geneva: World Health Organization.

Wright, J. (2007) 'Developing the public health workforce', in S. Griffiths and D.J. Hunter (eds) *New perspectives in public health* (2nd edn), Oxford: Radcliffe Publishing.

Notes

* Systematic literature review references.

** Scoping review references.

Index